"Why Do I Feel This Way?"

Natural Healing for Optimal Health and Relief from Moods and Depression

Suka Chapel-Horst, RN, PhD, QMHP

Brainworks Publishing

The purpose of this book is to educate. It is sold with the understanding that neither the publisher nor the author has any liability or responsibility for any injury caused or alleged to be caused directly or indirectly by the information contained in this book. While every effort has been made to insure its accuracy, the book's contents should not be construed as medical advice. To obtain medical advice on your individual health needs, please consult a qualified health care practitioner.

"WHY DO I FEEL THIS WAY?"
Natural Healing for Optimal Health and
Relief from Moods and Depression
By Suka Chapel-Horst, RN, PhD

Brainworks Publishing
638 Spartanburg Highway, Suite 70-175
Hendersonville, NC 28792

For orders and information go to:
www.BrainworksRecovery.com

While the author has made every effort to provide accurate telephone numbers and Internet addresses at the time of publication, neither the publisher nor the author assumes any responsibility for errors, or for changes that occur after publication.

ISBN: 0692268065
ISBN-13: 9780692268063

Library of Congress Control Number: 2013939393
Brainworks Publishing
Hendersonville North Carolina

DEDICATION

This book is dedicated to all those who joined the *PEERS OPTIMAL HEALTH PROGRAM* in Minneapolis and St. Paul, MN in the early 90's. Their successes paved the way for all those to come.

ACKNOWLEDGMENTS

Many, many thanks to my mentors, Joan Mathews-Larson, PhD, Julia Ross, MA, Hyla Cass, MD, Barbara Reed Stitt, PhD, William Walsh, PhD, and all the pioneers before them. My special thanks to my ever supportive husband, David Chapel Horst.

COVER ILLUSTRATION

My grandson, Tyler Hawk Richards, painted this picture when he was five years old in kindergarten. The original, 20" by 35", hangs on the wall in our home.

INTRODUCTION

This book is a first-step guide to optimal health. For most people, it will be all that's needed to achieve their health goals. The basic guidelines are pretty simple. The question is, "Do you care enough to do enough to achieve optimal health?" If your answer is "yes" then, this book is for you.

The concept of using micronutrient and amino acid therapy to restore health is new to many. Yet, ever-expanding knowledge obtained from neuroscience and biochemical research, plus over sixty years of direct experience, has proven the success of a natural approach for rebalancing brain chemistry and restoring optimal health, whenever possible.

For some, this book will mean not having to take prescription medications for moods and depression. For some this book will mean being able to come off their medications entirely, and for others, it will mean combining micronutrient and amino acid therapy with fewer and lower dosages of medications.

I have included *Resources for Daily Living*, which I originally published in *Onion Peelings – A Guide to Optimal Health* in 1992. Participants in my *Peers Optimal Health Program* in Minneapolis and St. Paul, MN, found these exercises to be very helpful for reducing stress and improving their quality of life. Although some of these exercises may seem unusual, at first, I urge you to try them. You will be pleasantly surprised, I promise.

There are many excellent resources available for those who want to go more deeply into this subject and we recommend them. However, for those who want the basic how-to's, this book is for you. My experience has been that most people will obtain excellent improvement in their health by just following these simple and effective guidelines.

I wish you good health, happy journeying, and profound peace.

Dr. Suka
May 1, 2013
Etowah, North Carolina

FORWARD

I grew up in Stoughton, Wisconsin, about 17 miles south of Madison. It was a typical, small Midwestern farming town. Well, not quite, because the town had a Norwegian heritage. Lefse, a Norwegian potato flat bread, was common fare. Lutefisk (a whitefish that smells like lye), floated in barrels of foul smelling brine that stood on sidewalks outside grocery store doors. As little girls, we pretended we were *Katrinka*, *Sigrid*, and *Olga*, speaking with a Norwegian accent, of course. Names ending with *son* were common, such as Anderson, Olson, and Knudson - my last name.

At our house, we ate all our meals together every day. Mother prepared simple, plain, and nutritious food. Breakfast was oatmeal, or eggs with bacon or ham, and orange juice. For dinner there was always a fruit salad, meat, potatoes, and a vegetable. Dessert was a small dish of ice cream or two homemade cookies, served about six o'clock every evening. Three or four times in the summer, we would go to a local drive-in that served scrumptious, freshly made, Bar-B-Q sandwiches and a root beer float and that's how most everyone in town ate. Food came fresh from the farms and orchards, filled with an abundance of healthy nutrients.

In my high school class of 103, there was only one fat person (we didn't use politically correct words then, such as obese.) and no one that we knew of had serious emotional or mental illnesses.

The mother of my friend, Barbara, was an alcoholic but no one knew that until much later. I liked being with her because she was such fun to be around. She loved to cook and fixed mouthwatering meals, three times a day. When I went over to Barbara's house, I almost always had to help her wash a stack of dishes, pots and pans, leftover from the previous meal before we were allowed to "go out and play".

Polio afflicted a number of my classmates, including another good friend, Susie, who developed serious scoliosis of the spine and had to wear a large, heavy back brace to school. Her brother's legs were crippled and he had to wear leg braces and use crutches.

Some of the high school kids had private parties where they drank beer and smoked cigarettes. One girl in my class became pregnant.

One day, a girlfriend and I took the train to Madison, about 17 miles away, just for the ride. In Madison, we each bought a pack of cigarettes (they didn't check our age) and smoked one on the train ride back home. It tasted horrible. I hid the pack in my bedroom and eventually threw all the cigarettes down the toilet, afraid of what my parents might do if I was caught. (I later took up smoking for nine years and loved every minute of it. I quit for several years and started again when I married a smoker. Three years after that I quit for good. Now, just the thought of smoking makes me sick but I admit, I enjoyed it while I did it.)

Stoughton was a safe town of 5,000 people who left their doors unlocked and where I was free to ride my bike everywhere, day or evening (but be in bed by 10 o'clock at night). I don't remember hearing of any criminal activity.

How life in the U.S. has changed. Yes, I had a protected childhood and was quite naive about life for a very long time. However, I was raised healthy and remain healthy today. Compare that simple life with today's demands, responsibilities, expectations, and stressors.

Beginning in the 1970's mountains of sugar and junk food infiltrated our culture, along with more pressures to excel, provide, and maintain a standard of life focused on acquiring *things*. Some couples dream of owning McMansions with granite countertops, stainless steel appliances, and two new cars in the driveway, plus one for the teen just learning to drive. Yet, for many, life isn't about the showy house and far-flung vacations, but rather about just keeping up, paying the bills, and staying out of bankruptcy.

Perhaps what has changed the most is the state of our health. The Infant Mortality Rate is the number of deaths-of-infants, under one year old, per 1,000 live births. This rate is often used as an indicator of the level of health in a country. Currently, the infant mortality rate in the U.S. ranks 34th from the top, in a list of all countries.

Life expectancy for the U.S. ranks 40th for the entire world. Obesity, infertility, diabetes, heart attacks, strokes, cancer, Alzheimer's, and other conditions are flaring out of sight. Sugar and junk fast-foods are the Standard American Diet (SAD). Alcohol and drug addiction continues, unabated. Depression is at an all time high. Chronic emotional and mental disorders are increasing, as is violence produced in response to SSRI antidepressants and anti-psychotic medications. [(See Appendix.)] In 2007-2008, one out of every five children and nine out of ten older Americans reported using at least one prescription drug in the past month. As the number of prescriptions medications have increased, our health has declined. Today...

We are more likely to take a pill than to fix dinner.

Restoring physical and emotional health is not rocket science. The answers are quite simple. Step off the treadmill of the typical American lifestyle and the Standard American Diet (SAD). Refuse junk food, soda pops, genetically modified organisms (GMO's), chemicals, preservatives, food colorings, processed foods, *and* the overuse and abuse of pharmaceutical medications.

We are fortunate to have neuroscience and biochemical research to support and educate us on how to accomplish a return to optimal health. Furthermore, we have our common sense. At our core most of us know that *natural* is natural.

Hippocrates said, "Let medicine be your food, and let food be your medicine". This is part of the Hippocratic Oath that physicians take upon graduation from medical school. It seems that most physicians were unconscious when they recited that part of the oath. It's up to us to remind them and to seek out qualified healthcare professionals who provide an integrative approach to wellness.

THE SOLUTION

We take charge of our health care. We employ our physicians, just the same as we employ an electrician or a book-keeper. We educate ourselves, inform our physicians, listen to and evaluate their suggestions, then WE DECIDE upon the best course of action. If we don't get what we want from a physician, we move on to the healthcare professionals we can depend upon.

Modern medicine is actually the alternative medicine.
Nature's medicine is what we are made of and nature knows best.

CONTENTS

CONGRATULATIONS

Where to begin? There is so much I'd like to share with you. Every day I run into people who are living with aches and pains, anxieties, the blahs or varying degrees of depression. They tell me about blood sugar and blood pressure levels that are out of control. Some tell me that they don't want to take medications so they continue to suffer without relief. Others say they are taking medications but are unhappy with the side effects. Some are afraid to get off their medications, fearing the return of earlier suffering. Many are drop-dead tired of yoyo dieting and weight gains. Some realize they are addicted to food, medications, work, exercise, the internet, TV, shopping, gambling, or relationships. They complain of insomnia, lack of energy, low motivation, or the opposite – being in high gear till they drop. Angry outbursts, irritability, self-doubt, helplessness and hopelessness are symptoms that are all too common.

Sometimes, if I happen to mention that there are safe and effective natural solutions, they just continue telling me more about their problems. I can read on their faces that they are stuck in mind-sets that foster and maintain poor health. I realize that they are not open to what I have to say, so I nod and listen, wish them well, and move on. And my heart hurts because I want so much to help, knowing that they could be far healthier and happier by using some simple strategies that could change their lives for the better.

But for those who choose to read this book, I congratulate you. I'm delighted to be able to offer you proven, simple, safe, and effective strategies for achieving optimal health.

For most of you, this book will be all you need to achieve optimal health. I have worked with hundreds of men and women who have completely recovered their health as a result of the information in this book. To be sure, there are some people who will benefit from more intensive help than this book offers. That's why, at the end of this book, I've listed the very best resources available today and I encourage you to contact them for help if it's indicated.

I believe that you are more interested in *getting* well than in *reading* about getting well. For that reason, I've attempted to keep this book as short and to-the-point as possible. The book is a first-step guide to optimal health, not the be-all end-all. However, for most of you, it's all you will need. Isn't that good news? So, let's begin.

THREE BODY TYPES

When I was in high school I learned about these body types and then forgot them until years later when they re-emerged while I was doing some research. When we understand the body type we are born with, it's easier to accept who we are, rather than attempting to be something we are not. Each body type is a gift, something to be proud of and to develop, using the strengths we are born with. This information can save a lot of grief by helping us to avoid trying to be something we are not. All body types are important and valued equally.

William Sheldon (1898-1977) was an American psychologist who spent his life observing all the varieties of human bodies. He taught at several universities and spent his career doing valuable research. As a child he was an avid observer of animals and birds, and as he grew up, this hobby turned into a strong ability to observe the human body. According to Dr. Sheldon, there are three body types, the endomorph, ectomorph, and mesomorph.

Below is a comparison between the three body types. While the labels stereotype people into three categories, they are still a useful tool for understanding one's makeup.

These body types are primarily motivated, on a physical level, by the muscular system, the digestive system or the nervous system. So, let's learn more about each of the body types.

Mesomorph – Muscular System

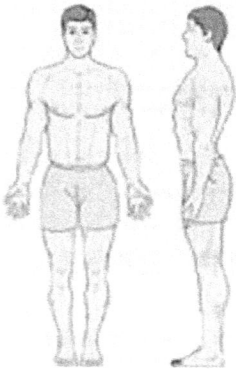

The mesomorph is dominated, primarily, by the muscular system. Touch a mesomorph and the skin will feel almost hot. They have a high metabolic rate which explains why they can eat more than others and not gain as much weight. FOOD MEANS FUEL to them. They tend to eat just what they need and burn off any excess with their high metabolism.

Mesomorphs tend to be very aware of where they are in space; call them grounded. You might say they walk firmly upon the earth. They seem to have physical substance and stability. When surprised or threatened, they tend to respond instinctively and quickly with ACTION. They think and feel later.

Grounded mesomorphs love how exercise makes them feel. Their muscles demand exercise. Even if they don't get regular exercise, they like to be active, and their bodies won't sit still for long. The mesomorph feels great when adrenalin is pumping and the brain is flooded with endorphins.

Mesomorphs usually gain weight when their muscles get flabby. Men tend to gain weight in their abdomen which is harder on the heart than excess weight on the thighs and hips. Often, mesomorphs get rid of excess weight just by exercising, which they enjoy anyway.

Endomorph – Digestive System

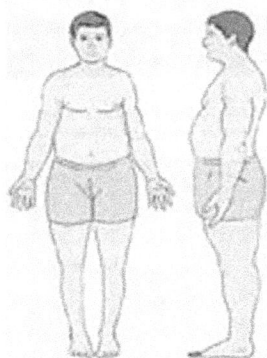

Endomorphs are physically dominated by their digestive system. They are usually round and have soft skin. Touch an endomorph and the skin will usually feel warm. Endomorphs are *very* sensitive to their surroundings and to people.

Their FEELINGS, both physical and emotional, respond first when they are surprised or threatened. Thinking and action follow the feelings.

Sometimes, the feelings are so strong endomorphs eat something, anything, just to become more comfortable. If too many of the feelings are uncomfortable, endomorphs sometimes learn to ignore their body signals and become almost unaware of their bodies from the neck down in order to avoid discomfort. They like life to be placid and comfortable. Discord feels very unpleasant to them.

For endormorphs, FOOD IS FUN, and because the digestive system is their predominant physical motivator, they can easily become overweight. In fact, the majority of chronically overweight people are endomorphs.

Endomorphs are highly sensitive. Layers of fat serve as protectors and barriers from outside negative influences. The *Resources for Daily Living* section of this book provides powerful tools for self-protection from negative stressors so that food doesn't have to be the solution. Endomorphs, especially, will benefit from these exercises.

Because of their desire for physical and emotional harmony, many endomorphs are not comfortable with strenuous exercise which requires large amounts of effort or short bursts of energy. It *feels* too *pushy* for them. They prefer walking, swimming and gentle sports such as golfing. Endomorphs are most happy when life is *flowing*. They seek the equilibrium of comfortably relaxed muscles and a gentle, easy flow of energy expenditure versus strenuous exercise.

Ectomorph – Nervous System

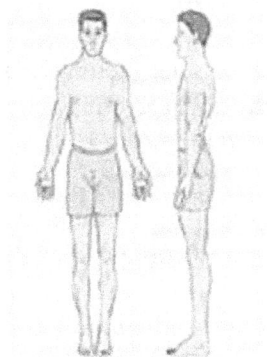

Ectomorphs are physically dominated by their nervous system. They usually have slender bodies and sometimes have sharp features. An ectomorphs's handshake will usually feel cool and their feet are often cold. When surprised or threatened, the ectomorph's first reaction is often to THINK about their response, acting second and lastly becoming aware of their feelings. They tend to be more controlled about their environment.

Ectomorphs enjoy FOOD but can often just TAKE IT OR LEAVE IT. Because of a normally low metabolism, ectomorphs tend to have yoyo weight swings of 10 to 20 pounds, but rarely carry large amounts of excess weight.

The wired ectomorphic body seems to have an abundance of energy even without exercise. Some like exercise and some "don't have time for it". Both gentle movement and strenuous exercise help to release the excess energy of this body.

PHYSICAL BODY TYPES SUMMARY

MESOMORPH

Muscular System	Action oriented
Firm bodies	Initiator
Strong muscles	Food is fuel
Hot blooded	Basketball
Grounded	Running
Instinctive	

ENDOMORPH

Digestive System	Placid
Round bodies	Reconciler
Soft skin	Food is fun
Warm blooded	Bowling
Sensitive	Walking
Feeling	

ECTOMORPH

Nervous System	Controlled
Slender bodies	Analyzer
Sharp features	Food is food
Cool blooded	Tennis
Wired	Skiing
Thinking	

Body Type Summary

Please remember, these body types are stereotyped for easier understanding of physical and emotional inclinations. I think it helps to know that some of our natural tendencies are motivated by the body itself, not just our minds. Above all, love your body type 'cause it's too late for a refund. Develop your body's potential and enjoy your unique and wonderful qualities.

Don't try to be someone you're not. We often spend our thinking time comparing ourselves to others and always coming out the loser. If only we could see our real self in the mirror. We would be amazed and awed at the wonderful and exciting being each one of us really is.

I see each and every one of you as a beautifully whole, healthy, and wonderful human being. I know you have the ability to achieve the optimal health you are capable of if you decide to put your heart into going for it. I'm supporting you all the way. Even as you read this book, I'm holding you in good health and wholeness in my heart.

THE UNFOLDING JOURNEY

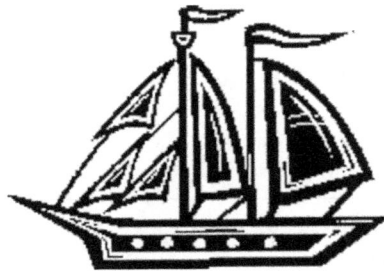

The brain does not recognize objects or concepts
for which there is no frame of reference.

When the Spaniards first anchored their galleons in the waters off the shores of South American in the 1500's, the natives didn't see them. Oh, their eyes saw the ships all right, but there was no concept of such large vessels in their consciousness. There were no mental brain cells for the images to connect with and therefore, the natives didn't see the ships.

We've all experienced the effect of being introduced to something new, something we knew nothing about in the past, and suddenly we hear about it, read about it, see it all around us. It was always there but we weren't interested enough to notice it before.

And so it is with the concept of how we respond to each other as human beings. Call it psychology or just plain relating to one another. Only recently in history have we become interested in communication styles, social behavior, and the quality of relationships. For most of history people married to meet survival needs including the gain of money, land ownership, and to have children to work the family business or farm (boys preferred). Girls were the means to the end. Working to survive and sexual attraction outweighed loving partnerships.

Yet, there are references to mental health in recorded history. Ancient manuscripts refer to a mental condition called "demon possession", now named schizophrenia. Every religion has exorcism rituals for "casting out the devils".

The Greek physician Hippocrates (460-370 BC) devised a psychological system called the Four Humours, relating to four body fluids. It's interesting to see how well thought out these were in light of today's psychology.

SANGUINE

Confidant	Late
Sociable	Forgetful
Creative	Sarcastic
Sensitive	Impulsive
Romantic	Talkative
Compassionate	Pleasure-seeking

CHOLERIC

Ambitious	Passion
Leader	Dominating
Highly organized or	Controlling
Highly disorganized	Mood swings
Aggressive	Deep sudden depression
Energy	

MELANCHOLIC

Introverted	Artistic
Thoughtful	Dramatic
Considerate	Perfectionists
Worried	Self reliant
On time	Independent
Highly creative	Preoccupied

PHLEGMATIC

Relaxed	Shy
Warm	Stable
Kind	Consistent
Lazy – sluggish	Rational
Accepting	Curious
Affectionate	Passive aggressive

The ideas of mental illness changed dramatically in the late 1800s, not so long ago, with the work of Sigmund Freud (1856-1939), Alfred Adler (1870-1937), and Carl Jung (1875-1961). The new thought was "it's all in the mind". A pioneer in the field of food and behavior and a friend of mine, Dr. Barbara Reed Stitt, coined a phrase describing this. She called it the "Ghost in the Machine" model of psychiatry. Suddenly, the mind and body became separate identities. Treatment for emotional and mental disorders was centered upon self-analysis, therapy, counseling and self-help programs. In some cases, therapy continues for years with varying levels of success and failure.

In 1955 the American Medical Association (AMA) and the World Health Organization (WHO) determined that mental illnesses were medical diseases in origin and in the 1960's schizophrenia, the old "demon" illness, was discovered to be the result of imbalanced brain chemistry, not childhood trauma or the environment one grew up in.

Excitedly, the pharmaceutical companies delved deeply into research looking for synthetic solutions to reorganize brain chemistry. (You can't patent and make money on natural solutions such as vitamins and minerals.) Hundreds of costly medicines have been, and continue to be, developed to provide relief for depression, anxiety, insomnia, obsessive compulsive disorders, and psychosis, for example. While these medicines have provided symptom-relief for many, the unwanted side effects and serious dangers have caused yet another set of diagnoses to be remedied, certainly a boon to the growing pharmaceutical industry.

In the 1970's the quickly growing specialty of psychiatry embraced new medicines designed to manipulate the biochemistry of mental illness while the unscientific and controversial psychiatric bible, Diagnostic and Statistical Manual of Mental Disorders (DSM5), expanded to define 200 mental conditions, a far cry from Hippocrates's Four Humours!

Meanwhile, therapists and counselors continue to focus on a psychological approach to wellness paying little attention to the underlying biochemical factors. So, current medical treatment is based upon using synthetic chemicals to relieve symptoms, while creating new symptoms due to side effects, while further distorting brain chemistry, coupled with talk-therapy which does nothing to correct the underlying biochemical cause of mental illness.

Many of these medications leave the patient feeling foggy and spacey, with low energy and motivation, decreased sex drive, weight gain and more. How effective can talk therapy be when focus, concentration, memory, and dampened emotions are running the show?

To add another dimension, 99% of addiction treatment centers, along with Alcoholics Anonymous (AA), which began in 1935, have never embraced the science behind addictions, still considering addictions to be mental illnesses, the separative "ghost in the machine" mentality. Ignoring the underlying biochemical cause of addictions entirely, they advocate recovery by will power, Higher Power, talk-therapy, and support, while steadfastly ignoring their 82% to 90% relapse rates.

In the summer of 2011 the American Society of Addiction Medicine (ASAM) officially announced that, indeed, addictions are caused by dysfunctional brain chemistry. Like "Johnny come late to the table", I've heard addiction physicians say, they now understand the underlying cause of addictions but they still don't have a cure. Whoa!

Biochemical research, from as early as the 1930's, has led to vast amounts of knowledge and experience in providing successful recovery methods for mental illness and addictions but mainstream medicine and psychiatry has failed to accept and adopt this information. What's going on?

TWO BRANCHES OF MEDICINE

Allopathic Medicine

Allopathic medicine is the traditional medical school curriculum. Crudely put, physicians are taught to diagnose, prescribe, and cut. Diagnosis is based upon meeting a certain number of criteria, or having a certain number of symptoms, which lead to a label, or disease condition. Once the disease label is determined, the condition is treated by prescriptions or surgery or both.

Pharmaceutical companies support medical schools with research grants. Non-medical, non-scientifically trained salespeople ("pharmaceutical reps") parrot the pharmaceutical company's line of information to "educate" physicians who don't have either the time, inclination, or expertise to look seriously and objectively at research studies, many of which are falsely performed and falsely reported. Many physicians are stealthily reimbursed for prescribing.

Medical students are not trained in nutritional biochemistry. They don't feel they have a need to understand this field because the pharmaceutical companies are doing the research and are happy to supply them with their synthetic medicines.

As neuroscience sheds increasingly more light on brain chemistry, allopathic physicians have been forced to consider the effects of biochemistry, however, being uneducated about natural methods of correcting brain chemistry, they have increasingly relied even more on the synthetic products of the pharmaceutical companies. Today pharmaceutical companies are buying up supplement companies and making synthetic "natural" supplements.

Orthomolecular Medicine

Orthomolecular is a term that comes from the word "ortho", which is Greek for "correct" or "right," and "molecule," which is the simplest structure that displays the characteristics of a compound. So it literally means the "right molecule."

Two-time Nobel Prize winner, and molecular biologist, Linus Pauling, Ph.D., coined the term "Orthomolecular" in his 1968 article *"Orthomolecular Psychiatry"* in the journal "Science."

Instead of diagnosing people with disease labels and treating a disease, orthomolecular physicians look for the underlying cause, or chemical imbalance, that exists within the body and brain. Treatment consists of rebalancing the brain/body with the natural biochemical components, building blocks, of which it is made.

Correcting biochemical imbalances through the use of natural substances is extremely effective, practical, safe, creates no side effects, and costs very little. Because the pharmaceutical companies can't make money on natural substances, they use the identical research to create *synthetic* products that *resemble* the natural substances. These drugs do, sometimes, relieve the symptoms, but... they create side effects and serious life-threatening reactions while further distorting the underlying chemical imbalances. Note the following.

Prescription medications, taken as directed, are the fourth leading cause of hospital *deaths* topped only by heart disease, cancer and stroke.[1] The *death* rate from prescription drugs, taken as directed, in 2008 was *three times greater* than from all illicit drugs combined.[2]

I find it disturbing that the American Medical Association has banned orthomolecular research from their medical journals and from government owned medical libraries. Unfortunately, government driven universities are not eager to provide grants for research into natural methods of biochemical recovery, for obvious reasons.

That said, there is an abundance of research information available through independent sources. Just put *orthomolecular, functional,* or *integrative medicine* into the internet and you'll find a wealth of scientific and evidence based information. Like the ship that wasn't seen by the South American natives, once you begin looking for this information, you'll easily find it.

Allopathic medicine works from the outside in.
Orthomolecular medicine works from the inside out.

SUMMARY

Allopathic medicine is based on organ systems with physicians specializing in different systems. Orthomolecular medicine views the body as one interdependent system so that treatment is directed at rebalancing and correcting the chemistry of the entire system.

Fortunately, the field of Integrative and Holistic Medicine is growing and bringing together the best of ancient and modern, eastern and western, allopathic and orthomolecular medicine.

Now you have a frame of reference for the rest of the material in this book.

Happy sailing.

1 Florida Medical Examiners Commission, 2008
2 Federal: Agency for Healthcare Research & Quality, The National Academy of Sciences' Institute of Medicine, 2008

PART ONE

Self-Testing

JINX IN THE BOX

In the last chapter I talked about the concept of the *"ghost in the machine"*, or the mind, as being separate from the body. If this is not true, are we, then, just a product of the brain? Nothing more? Of course not. I like to explain it this way.

Suppose you are a NASCAR race driver, or a driving instructor. You're ready to go. You slide into the driver's seat, turn on the ignition, and nothing happens because the car has no gas in the tank, no air in the tires, no water in the radiator, and no oil in the crank case. How far are you going to go? There's nothing wrong with the driver but if the vehicle isn't operable, this fine driver isn't going anywhere.

In the same manner, we are beautiful souls at the mercy of our physical vehicle, the brain. Fortunately, our brains are more flexible than cars. The brain allows us to get away without fueling it frequently or properly for awhile. The body's flexibility lulls us into ignoring its needs until it can no longer adapt. That's when we take notice that some things are not going right. Cars sputter, jerk, shake, and make loud noises. Humans experience anxiety, panic, frequent colds, aches and pains, difficulty breathing, insomnia, depression, and cravings. These are just a few of the notices humans get from the overstressed and undernourished brain.

So, maintaining balanced brain chemistry is the same as putting fuel, air, water, and oil into a car. The brain is the box and the jinx in the box is imbalanced brain chemistry that keeps the driver, or soul, from its full potential or from having optimal health.

DIVING WITHIN

Before putting together a plan for recovery, it's obvious that we need to find out what is going on under the hood of our vehicle. The following ten tests[1] will help to answer the question, *"Could I have this condition?"* Many of the symptoms are the same from test to test, therefore, it's important to take all the tests to get a complete picture.

1. Follow the directions given with each test.
2. Answer the questions according to how you feel NOW, not how you felt in the past.

---

1   These tests have been derived from leading experts in the field of health and wellness, including William Crook, MC, Julia Ross, MA, Joan Mathews-Larson, PhD, George Kroker, MD, and William Walsh, PhD.

3. If you are questioning whether a symptom is true for you, it probably isn't important. If you have a symptom, you know it. It's experienced frequently or most of the time. We all have some symptoms, some of the time but they are not a problem.

4. Write down your scores at the end of each test, and also on the Total Accumulated Score sheet in Chapter 14.

Suggestions for follow-up are given at the end of each test. In some cases, if your scores indicate a need for further testing, you will be advised to see a health care provider. Many of these conditions can be effectively reversed with an appropriate nutritional diet and the right micronutrients and food supplements.

In case you may be inclined to skip these tests and just dive into repair, please think again. If any of these underlying issues are present and not addressed, recovery will be uncertain, at best.

CARBOHYDRATE ADDICTION TEST

It's difficult to avoid the bad (simple) carbohydrates. Sugar, in many forms, is found in all processed foods, very often as a first or second ingredient. Excess sugar is a poison, four times more addictive than cocaine.

American's love affair with the "whites" (flour, rice, pasta, potatoes, etc.) continues to grow. And now, the food industry is regularly including chemicals in foods that stimulate the appetite. 35.7% of Americans are obese (20% over normal weight) and 68% are overweight (20 or more pounds above normal weight).

11.3% of people over age 20 and 26.9% of people over age 65 have diabetes and the number is climbing as Americans make sugar and simple carbohydrates their number-one foods of choice.

While most of us consume some level of sugars, and other simple carbohydrates, not everyone is addicted to it, though most are. An addiction creates symptoms of dis-ease in all its forms. Take this test to find out if you are addicted to simple carbohydrates.

_____ 1. When eating sweets, starches, or snack foods, do you find it hard to stop?

_____ 2. At a restaurant, do you eat several rolls or bread before the meal is served?

_____ 3. While eating carbohydrates, do you ever feel out of control?

_____ 4. Does your diet consist mainly of breads, pastas, starchy vegetables, fast foods, and/or sweets?

_____ 5. Do you ever hide food or eat food secretly?

_____ 6. Do you binge on snack foods, candy, or fast foods?

_____ 7. Does eating a sweet snack lift your spirits?

_____ 8. Do you feel hungry and unsatisfied after a meal no matter how much you eat?

_____ 9. Do you feel sleepy or groggy after a high-carbohydrate meal (i.e., breads, potatoes, pastas, dessert)?

_____ 10. Which would you prefer:

_____ breaded fish	or	_____ baked fish
_____ potato	or	_____ broccoli
_____ sandwich	or	_____ salad
_____ chips	or	_____ raw nuts
_____ cookie	or	_____ strawberries
_____ cracker	or	_____ raw vegetables
_____ spaghetti	or	_____ steak

(For question 10, consider your response a "yes" if you checked more items in the left-hand column than in the right-hand column.)

Total the number of "yes" responses to these ten questions. Then determine which of the following categories you fit into:

TOTAL SCORE: _____

1-2 Doubtful Addiction,

3-4 Mild Addiction,

5-6 Moderate Addiction

7-10 Severe Addiction

If your score is over 5, you will benefit by restricting your carbohydrates to fifty to seventy-five grams daily. Follow the LOW CARBOHYDRATE FOOD PLAN in Chapter 23 for three to four weeks, then shift to the OPTIMAL HEALTH FOOD PLAN.

In almost all cases, your weight will shift toward normal in a healthy and gradual manner. Many symptoms of dis-ease will simply disappear.

Adapted from *Seven Weeks to Sobriety – Joan Mathews Larson, Ph.D.*

CANDIDA

30 million plus people suffer from an *overgrowth* of *candida* and that's only the number in North America. Roughly half the world's population will suffer from a candida-related condition in their lifetime.

Candida is a type of yeast fungus normally found among the balance of "good" and "bad" bacteria in a healthy person's digestive system. It lives in 80% of the human population without causing harmful effects. Usually kept in check by the intestine's friendly flora, lactobacilli acidophilus, bifidophilus and others, when there is an overgrowth many symptoms can develop. Because the yeast lives on sugar, it will cause irresistible cravings making it difficult to stop addictions to alcohol, drugs, and sweet foods.

The person with candida overgrowth may be walking through life quite ill with the following experiences:

✓ All laboratory tests come back "normal".
✓ You're being treated for various ailments whose symptoms return when the medication is finished, possibly with additional side effects and no resolution.
✓ You've been told your symptoms are "psychological".
✓ You are misdiagnosed and incorrectly treated, worsening your health challenges.

An overgrowth of Candida yeast blocks proper digestion and elimination. It robs the body of vitamins, minerals and other nutrients from both food and supplements. It spreads from the gut to genitals, oral cavities and mucous membranes, pouring toxins into the blood and eventually affecting various organs in the body. In short, *candida eats what you eat, and when there is no nutrition left, it nourishes itself on your muscles and bones*. Where it can't eat, it causes deterioration.

Therefore, candida is tied into many of our chronic ailments and can create a miserable situation for its host if not caught and treated. Enough said.

CANDIDA

Section A: History

_____1. Have you taken tetracycline's or other antibiotics for acne for 1 month (or longer)? Give yourself 35 points

_____2. Have you at any time in your life taken broad-spectrum antibiotics or other antibacterial medications for respiratory, urinary or other infections for two months or longer, or in shorter courses four or more times in one year? 35 points

_____3. Have you taken a broad-spectrum antibiotic drug-even in a single dose? 6 points

_____4. Have you at any time in your life, been bothered by persistent prostatitis, vaginitis, or other problems affecting your reproductive organs? 25 points

_____5. Are you bothered by memory or concentration problems? Do you sometimes feel spaced out? 20 points

_____6. Do you feel "sick all over" yet, in spite of visits to many different physicians, the causes have not been found? 20 points

_____7. Have you been pregnant...2 or more times? 5 points ...one time? 3 points

_____8. Have you taken birth control pills... for more than two years? 15 points ... for six months to two years? 8 points

_____9. Have you taken steroids orally, by injection or inhalation... for more than two weeks? 15 points ....for two weeks or less? 6 points

_____10. Does exposure to perfumes, insecticides, and other chemicals provoke moderate to severe symptoms? 20 points .... mild symptoms? 5 points

_____11. Does tobacco smoke really bother you? 10 points

_____12. Are your symptoms worse on damp, muggy days, or in moldy places? 20 points

_____13. Have you had athlete's foot, ring worm, jock itch, or other chronic fungal infections of the skin or nails? Have such infections been... severe or persistent? 20 points... mild to moderate? 10 points

_____14. Do you crave sugar? 10 points

TOTAL SCORE, Section A _____

Section B: Major Symptoms

Does not apply=0 points

Mild or occasional=3 points

Moderate or frequent=6 points

Severe or disabling=9 points

_____ 1. Fatigue or lethargy

_____ 2. Feeling drained

_____ 3. Depression or manic depression

_____ 4. Numbness, burning or tingling

_____ 5. Headache

_____ 6. Muscle aches

_____ 7. Muscle weakness or paralysis

_____ 8. Pain and/or swelling in joints

_____ 9. Abdominal pain

_____10. Constipation and/or diarrhea

_____11. Bloating, belching or intestinal gas

_____12. Vaginal burning, itching or discharge

_____13. Prostatitis

_____14. Impotence

_____15. Loss of sexual desire or feeling

_____16. Endometriosis or infertility

_____17. Cramps and/or other menstrual irregularities

_____18. Premenstrual tension

_____19. Attacks of anxiety or crying

_____20. Cold hands or feet, low body temperature

_____21. Hypothyroidism

_____22. Shaking or irritable when hungry

_____23. Cystitis or interstitial cystitis (bladder inflammation)

TOTAL SCORE, Section B _____

Section C, Other Symptoms

Does not apply = 0 points

Mild or occasional = 1 point

Moderate or frequent = 2 points

Severe or disabling = 3 points

_____ 1. Drowsiness, including inappropriate drowsiness

_____ 2. Irritability

_____ 3. Uncoordinated

_____ 4. Frequent mood swings

_____ 5. Insomnia

_____ 6. Dizziness/loss of balance

_____ 7. Pressure above ears... feeling of head swelling

_____ 8. Sinus problems... tenderness of cheekbones or forehead

_____ 9. Tendency to bruise easily

_____10. Eczema, itching eyes

_____11. Psoriasis

_____12. Chronic hives (urticaria)

_____13. Indigestion or heartburn

_____14. Sensitivity to milk, wheat, corn or other common foods

_____15. Mucus in stools

_____16. Spots in front of eyes or erratic vision

_____17. Burning or tearing eyes

_____18. Recurrent infections or fluid in ears

_____19. Ear pain or deafness

TOTAL SCORE, Section C _____

Score, Section A _____

Score, Section B _____

Score, Section C _____

GRAND TOTAL Score _____

RESULTS

If your score is MORE THAN 180 in women and MORE THAN 140 in men, systemic yeast is **almost certainly** present.

If your score is MORE THAN 120 in women and MORE THAN 90 in men, systemic yeast is **probably** present.

If your score is MORE THAN 60 in women and MORE THAN 40 in men, systemic yeast is **possibly** present.

With scores LESS THAN 60 in women and LESS THAN 40 in men, systemic yeast is **less likely** to cause health problems.

This questionnaire is taken from *The Yeast Connection Handbook*, by William G. Crook, MD. 1999

Candida can sometimes be cured with non-prescription supplements, however you may need to use a prescription such as Diflucan, especially if you have a very bad case. It's important to eliminate junk foods, sugars, pastas, and white flour products from the diet, and to take food supplements, including a B vitamin complex. Homeopathic products can be helpful, as well.

FOOD ALLERGIES

Whole grain wheat bread is good for us, right? Maybe. Maybe we eat it as toast or cereal for breakfast, in a sandwich for lunch, a late afternoon beer or two, and as bread with dinner. We don't associate our fatigue or insomnia with healthy bread, but these and other symptoms we're experiencing may be the result of an allergy to wheat or gluten. We won't know until we test for allergies. The test is simple and can be done at home.

Allergies are far more common than most people think and are the cause of so many symptoms. The good news is that once the allergy is detected, by eliminating the offending food from one's diet, the symptoms are relieved. No more suffering and no more prescription medications to cover up the symptoms. (One can occasionally eat the offending food later.) The most common allergens are 1) wheat and its cousins - rye, barley, and oats, and 2) cow's milk products including milk, cheese or anything else made from the modern cow. Runners-up are soy and the nightshade family (tomatoes, peppers, white potatoes, eggplant, and tobacco). Runners-up, especially for children, are chocolate, corn, peanuts, eggs, oranges, and foods high in salicylates like apples[1]

Do you crave it? Eat it daily? Don't want to give it up? These are clues. Listed below are some allergy related disorders.

- Attention deficit
- Bronchial asthma
- Bronchitis
- Chronic diarrhea
- Chronic fatigue syndrome
- Depression
- Headaches (migraine and non-migraine)
- Hyperactivity
- Insomnia
- Learning disorders
- Sleep disorders
- Tension-fatigue syndrome

ALLERGY SYMPTOMS Check all symptoms that apply to you.

_____   Irritability

_____   Angry outbursts

_____   Glum lethargy

_____   Teariness

_____   Hyperactivity

_____   Stress

_____   Depression

_____   Asthma

_____   Sore throat

_____   Earaches

_____   Stuffy nose

_____   Postnasal drip

_____   Constipation

_____   Diarrhea

_____   Stomachache

_____   Bloat

_____   Gas

_____   Reflux

_____   Heartburn

_____   Low energy

_____   Sleepiness (especially right after meals)

_____   Joint pain

_____   Achiness

_____   Poor concentration

_____   Addictive cravings for the allergy food or for sweets

_____ **TOTAL SYMPTOM SCORE** A high score may indicate allergies.

INSTRUCTIONS

1. Complete the first four questions.
2. In Question Five, Food Questionnaire, **circle any foods** you listed in Question Three.
3. Women only: In Question Five **circle any foods** you listed in Question Four.
4. In Question Five, **circle any heading** above a section that contains foods eaten six or seven days per week.

SCREENING TEST FOR FOOD ALLERGIES

1. List a typical day's meals and snacks:

BREAKFAST   LUNCH   DINNER   SNACKS

_____

_____

_____

_____

_____

2. List your three most favorite foods that you eat regularly.

_____

3. Do you crave or binge on any foods: If so, which ones?

_____

4. (For women) Do you crave or binge on foods premenstrually? If so, which ones?

_____

5. Food Questionnaire
How many days in one week do you eat the following foods: (Write the number of days on the line following the food.)

WHEAT/YEAST

Bread	____	Spaghetti	____
Rolls	____	Casseroles	____
Muffins	____	Pizza	____
Sandwiches	____	Breakfast cereal	____
Bagels	____	Crackers	____
Pasta	____	Cookies	____
Macaroni	____	Canned soup	____
Noodles	____	Pastries	____

CORN

Popcorn	____	Cornflakes	____
Lunch meat	____	Corn (vegetable)	____
Tacos	____	Pancake syrup	____

OTHER GRAINS

Rice	____	Other	____
Oatmeal	____		

DAIRY

Milk	____	Margarine	____
Cheese	____	Butter	____
Yogurt	____	Cream cheese	____
Ice cream	____	Cottage cheese	____
Coffee creamer	____		

EGGS

Scrambled, omelet, etc.	____	French toast	____
Mayonnaise	____		

MISCELLANEOUS

Vinegar	____	Prunes	____
Salad dressing	____	Ketchup	____

Mushrooms	____	Mustard	____
Soy sauce	____	Peanuts	____
Raisons	____	Other nuts	____
Dates	____		

DESSERT

Jell-0	____	Sweet 'N Low	____
Jelly/jam	____	Equal	____
		NutraSweet	____

BEEF

| Beef roast | ____ | Steak | ____ |
| Hamburger | ____ | | |

PORK

| Ham | ____ | Sausage | ____ |
| Bacon | ____ | Pork chops | ____ |

OTHER PROTEIN

Chicken	____	_____	____
Turkey	____	_____	____
Fish	____	Soy/tofu	____
_____	____	Hot dogs	____

BEVERAGES

Diet soda	____	Coffee	____
Alcoholic beverages	____	Tea	____
Soda	____	Fruit juice	____

SNACKS

| Potato chips | ____ | Chocolate | ____ |

FRUIT

Apples	____	Grapes	____
Bananas	____	Pineapple	____
Oranges	____	Other:	
Pears	____	_____	____
Melon	____	_____	____
Grapefruit	____		

VEGETABLES

Tomato	____	Broccoli	____
Green pepper	____	Cabbage/coleslaw	____
Peas	____	Cauliflower	____
Green beans	____	Other:	____
Other beans:		_____	____
_____	____	Lettuce salads	____
Carrots	____	Potatoes/French fries	____
Celery	____		

SPICES

Onion	____	Ginger	____
Garlic	____	Parsley	____
Pepper	____	Oregano	____
Dry mustard	____	Cinnamon	____
Basil	____	Mint	____
Paprika	____	Other:_____	____
Rosemary	____	_____	____

This self-screening test was designed by George Kroker, M.D.

INSTRUCTIONS repeated

1. Complete the first four questions.
2. In Question Five, Food Questionnaire, **circle any foods** you listed in Question Three.
3. Women only: In Question Five **circle any foods** you listed in Question Four.
4. In Question Five, **circle any heading** above a section that contains foods eaten six or seven days per week.

LIST THE FOODS YOU HAVE CIRCLED IN QUESTION FIVE

_____

_____

_____

The foods you have circled and listed above are the ones most likely to trigger addictive cravings and delayed allergic reactions. Allergic reactions occur within minutes to forty eight hours after eating the offending food. That's why we wait 72 hours before testing a second food.

The most effective test for food allergies is the elimination diet. This test is fully explained in Chapter 24.

1 *The Mood Cure* by Julia Ross, MA, p 137

7

HYPOGLYCEMIA

Hypoglycemia, or low blood sugar, is an abnormally diminished amount of glucose in the blood. The term literally means "low sugar blood". It can produce a variety of symptoms and effects but the principal problems arise from an inadequate supply of glucose to the brain, resulting in impairment of function.

Effects can range from mild mental and emotional experiences of depression, discontent and indifference to the world around one to more serious issues such as seizures, unconsciousness, and (rarely) permanent brain damage or death.

SYMPTOMS OF HYPOGLYCEMIA

Place a check mark in front of any or all the symptoms you frequently experience.

_____ Nervousness

_____ Anxiety

_____ Irritability

_____ Indecisiveness

_____ Exhaustion

_____ Weakness

_____ Rapid pulse

_____ Sweating

_____ Heart palpitations

_____ Depression

_____ Internal trembling

_____ Forgetfulness

_____ Headaches

_____ Hunger

_____ Sighing or yawning

_____ Craving for sweetness or alcohol

_____ Faintness

_____ Dizziness

_____ Uncoordinated

_____ Double vision

_____ Drowsiness   _____ Blurred vision

_____ Leg cramps   _____ Tremor

_____ Unprovoked anxieties   _____ Seizures

_____ Insomnia   _____ Suicidal thoughts

_____ Frustration   _____ Loss of consciousness

_____ Crying spells   _____ Numbness

_____ Mental confusion   _____ Muscle twitching or jerking

_____ Abnormal behavior   _____ Itching and crawling skin sensations

_____ Constant worrying   _____ Tingling sensation around the mouth

HYPOGLYCEMIA TOTAL SCORE _____

If you tested positive for several of these symptoms, your health will rapidly improve by getting off sugar products and low carbohydrates, including all junk, processed, and white foods. (See Chapter 23.)

If you tested positive for a Carbohydrate Addiction (Chapter 4), you are most likely also hypoglycemic. 95% to 100% of alcoholics are hypoglycemic, but then, so are most Americans.

Hypoglycemia creates strong cravings for sugar which is in all processed food, junk food, and sodas. Food cravings, obesity and diabetes are directly related to hypoglycemia. Alcohol rapidly converts to sugar. Tobacco is cured in sugar. With the aid of a good supplement and nutritional program, this condition can be reversed.

HYPOTHYROIDISM

The thyroid gland makes two primary hormones, T3 and T4. The T stands for the amino acid Tyrosine and the 3 and 4 stand for the number of iodine molecules in each hormone. These two hormones ignite every cell of your body and brain by activating its genetic coding. Without proper thyroid function, the neurotransmitters can't alter your moods effectively.

Everyone should have a thyroid function test on a regular basis. Certainly, if your thyroid function is less than normal and left untreated, proper nutrition and supplementation, while helpful, will not provide you the rewards you hope for.

There are three kinds of thyroid diseases. Graves Disease and hyPERthyroidism. However, the most common thyroid malfunction is hyPOthyroidism. If your moods, depression, or other symptoms are caused by hypothyroidism, you'll want to know about it and correct the condition.

RISK FACTORS FOR HYPOTHYROIDISM INCLUDE (BUT ARE NOT LIMITED TO):

* Family history of thyroid disease
* History of another autoimmune disease
* Had a baby in the past nine months
* History of miscarriage

SYMPTOMS OF HYPOTHYROIDISM

Check all symptoms you frequently experience.

_____ Gaining weight inappropriately

_____ Unable to lose weight with diet/exercise

_____ Constipated, sometimes severely

_____ Hypothermia/low body temperature (Feel cold when others feel hot, need extra sweaters, etc.)

_____ Fatigued, exhausted

_____ Run down, sluggish, lethargic

_____ Hair is coarse and dry, breaking, brittle, falling out

_____ Skin is coarse, dry, scaly, and thick

_____ Hoarse or gravely voice

_____ Puffiness and swelling around the eyes and face

_____ Pains, aches in joints, hands and feet

_____ Carpal-tunnel syndrome

_____ Irregular menstrual cycles (longer, or heavier, or more frequent)

_____ Trouble conceiving a baby

_____ Depressed

_____ Restless

_____ Moods change easily

_____ Feelings of worthlessness

_____ Difficulty concentrating

_____ Feelings of sadness

_____ Losing interest in normal daily activities

_____ More forgetful lately

_____ Hair is falling out

_____ Can't seem to remember things

_____ No sex drive

_____ Getting more frequent infections, that last longer

_____ Snoring more lately

_____ Have or may have sleep apnea

_____ Shortness of breath and tightness in the chest

_____ Feel the need to yawn to get oxygen

_____ Eyes feel gritty and dry

_____ Eyes feel sensitive to light

_____ Eyes get jumpy/tics in eyes creating dizziness/vertigo and headaches

_____ Strange feelings in neck or throat

_____ Tinnitus (ringing in ears)

_____ Recurrent sinus infections

_____ Vertigo

_____ Lightheadedness

_____ Menstrual cramps

TOTAL SCORE _____

If you have several of these symptoms, inform your healthcare provider, and get a lab test, and medication if appropriate. Natural thyroid supplementation does not usually provide consistent dependable quality. We recommend prescription medication which is inexpensive and works very well.

LABORATORY TESTING: I recommend getting TSH, Free T3 and Free T4 testing. Your physician may not want to do the Free T3 and Free T4 tests. They are far more accurate than the T3 and T4. If your physician refuses, see testing resources in Appendix C.

ADRENAL INSUFFICIENCY

The adrenal glands are about the size of an almond, and sit on top of the kidneys. These glands are extremely important and affect the way we think and feel. They affect how fats and carbohydrates are used and are a factor in fat and protein metabolism. These glands affect blood-sugar regulation and proper cardiovascular and gastrointestinal functions.

The adrenal glands are responsible for helping the body cope with stress and survive through stress. They allow the body to deal with stress from every possible source whether it is job related, or from injury, disease, relationship problems or just the stresses of everyday life. Listed below are some of the lifestyles that can contribute to adrenal fatigue.

LIFESTYLE STRESSORS

_____ College students

_____ Single parenting

_____ Self-employed business owner

_____ Alternating shift work (improper sleeping schedule)

_____ Disease

_____ Death of close friend or family member

_____ Drug or alcohol abuse

_____ Head trauma

_____ Loss of job

_____ Moving to a new home or city

_____ Relationship issues

_____ Serious burns (even severe sunburn)

_____ Severe emotional trauma (death or being the caregiver of a sick individual)

_____ Work pressures

TOTAL NUMBER OF STRESSORS _____

SYMPTOMS OF ADRENAL INSUFFICIENCY

_____ **Hypoglycemia** (See Chapter 7)

_____ Dehydration

_____ Weight loss

_____ Disorientation

_____ Weakness

_____ Tiredness

_____ Dizziness

_____ Low blood pressure that falls further when standing

_____ Muscle aches

_____ Nausea

_____ Vomiting

_____ Diarrhea

_____ Pupils that don't contract

_____ Steroid drugs

_____ Type II diabetes (which is an adrenal issue)

TOTAL SCORE _____

If you think you may have adrenal insufficiency, contact your holistic health practitioner, your chiropractor, acupuncturist, or nutritionist for testing. Acupuncturists have been successfully treating adrenal insufficiency for thousands of years.

For the location of recommended laboratory testing facilities go to Resources C.

ALCOHOL SCREENING

Developed in 1971, the **MICHIGAN ALCOHOL SCREENING TEST, (MAST)**, is one of the oldest and most accurate alcohol screening tests available. It identifies dependent drinkers with up to 98% accuracy.

The MAST test is a simple, self-scoring test that helps assess if you have a drinking problem. Answer "yes" or "no" to the following:

1. ___ Yes ___ No   Do you feel you are a normal drinker ("normal" is defined as drinking as much as, or less than, most other people)?

2. ___ Yes ___ No   Have you ever awakened the morning after drinking the night before and found that you could not remember a part of the evening?

3. ___ Yes ___ No   Does any near relative or close friend ever worry or complain about your drinking?

4. ___ Yes ___ No   Can you stop drinking without difficulty after one or two drinks?

5. ___ Yes ___ No   Do you ever feel guilty about your drinking?

6. ___ Yes ___ No   Have you ever attended a meeting of Alcoholics Anonymous (AA)?

7. ___ Yes ___ No   Have you ever gotten into physical fights when drinking?

8. ___ Yes ___ No   Has drinking ever created problems between you and a near relative or close friend?

9. ___ Yes ___ No   Has any family member or close friend gone to anyone for help about your drinking?

10. ___ Yes ___ No   Have you ever lost friends because of your drinking?

11. ___ Yes ___ No   Have you ever gotten into trouble at work because of drinking?

12. ___ Yes ___ No   Have you ever lost a job because of drinking?

13. ___ Yes ___ No   Have you ever neglected your obligations, family, or work for two or more days in a row because you were drinking?

14. ___ Yes ___ No   Do you drink before noon fairly often?

15. ___ Yes ___ No   Have you ever been told you have liver trouble, such as cirrhosis?

16. ___ Yes ___ No   After heavy drinking, have you ever had delirium tremens (DTs), severe shaking, visual or auditory (hearing) hallucinations?

17. ___ Yes ___ No   Have you ever gone to anyone for help about your drinking?

18. ___ Yes ___ No   Have you ever been hospitalized because of drinking?

19. ___ Yes ___ No   Has your drinking ever resulted in your being hospitalized in a mental health facility?

20. ___ Yes ___ No   Have you ever gone to any doctor, social worker, clergy person, or mental health clinic for help with any emotional problem in which drinking was part of the problem?

21. ___ Yes ___ No   Have you been arrested more than once for driving under the influence of alcohol?

22. ___ Yes ___ No   Have you ever been arrested, or detained by an official for a few hours, because of other behavior while drinking?

SCORE one point each if you answered "no" to questions 1 and 4. _____

SCORE one point each if you answered "yes" to questions 2, 3, and 5 through 22. _____

TOTAL SCORE _____

A **total score of six or more** indicates hazardous drinking or alcohol dependence and further evaluation by a healthcare professional is recommended. This includes reversing the condition immediately by getting the appropriate help.

See Appendix B - Recovery Resources that focus on restoring biochemical imbalances. Also, read the book *How to Quit Drinking For Good and Feel Good – The NEW Alcoholism Story* by Suka Chapel-Horst, RN, PhD. Available on the web site www.AriseAlcoholRecovery.com.

11

PYROLOURIA

Pyroluria is the result of a genetically-caused over-production of a group of chemicals called kyrptopyrroles. These pyrroles bind with B_6 and zinc and dump them into the urine which is then excreted from the body creating emotional disaster. A high incidence of Pyrrole Disorder is found in individuals on the autism spectrum, individuals with anxiety disorder, depression, obsessive-compulsive disorder, schizophrenia, bipolar disorder, Aspergers, AD(H)D, and alcoholism (44%). However, pyroluria is quickly and easily corrected when diagnosed.

MAJOR INDICATIONS

Check "yes" or "no" for each question below.

YES	NO	
____	____	Do you sunburn easily? Do you have fair or pale skin?
____	____	Do you tend to avoid stressful situations?
____	____	Do you have poor dream recall or only exciting dreams (nightmares)?
____	____	Is it hard to recall what you've just read?
____	____	Are your eyes sensitive to bright lights?
____	____	Do you get frequent colds or infections?
____	____	Are there white spots/flecks on your fingernails?
____	____	Are you prone to acne, eczema, or psoriasis?
____	____	Do you have stretch marks on your skin?

____   ____   Do you prefer not to eat breakfast or even experience light nausea in the morning?

____   ____   Are there severe mood problems, mental illness, or alcoholism in your family?

SCORE YES ANSWERS _____

INDICATIONS THAT ARE OCCASIONALLY PRESENT

YES   NO

____   ____   Do you have a reduced amount of head hair or do you have prematurely gray hair?

____   ____   Are you becoming more of a loner as you age?

____   ____   Have you been anxious, fearful, or felt a lot of inner tension since childhood?

____   ____   If you are over age 16, do you have bouts of depression and/or nervous exhaustion?

____   ____   Do you have headaches?

____   ____   Did you reach puberty earlier or later than normal?

____   ____   Do you sneeze in sunlight?

____   ____   Do loud noises bother you?

____   ____   Do you prefer the company of one or two close friends rather than a gathering of friends?

____   ____   Have you noticed a sweet smell (fruity odor) to your breath or sweat when ill or stressed? (Rare symptom)

____   ____   Do you have a poor appetite or a poor sense of taste? Do you enjoy spicy food?

____   ____   Do you have any upper abdominal or spleen pain? As a child, did you get a "stitch" in your side when you ran? (1 in 10 have this symptom.)

____   ____   Do your knees crack or ache?

____   ____   Are you anemic? (1 in 10 have this symptom)

____   ____   Are you easily upset (internally) by criticism?

____   ____   Do you have frequent mood swings?

____   ____   Do you tend to carry any excess fat in your lower extremities rather than evenly distributed around your body (a pear-shaped figure)?

SCORE YES ANSWERS _____

If you have any of the disorders listed at the beginning of this chapter and you checked "yes" to five or more of the MAJOR INDICATIONS and *some* of the OCCASIONALLY PRESENT questions, you may benefit from a Pyrrole urine test.

© 2013 *This questionnaire, originally developed by Carl Pfeiffer, PhD., has been updated by Suka Chapel-Horst, RN, PhD, in consultation with William J. Walsh, PhD.*

This condition, if present, is 100% correctable with the proper micronutrients. Recovery can occur in a few weeks.

For the location of recommended laboratory testing facilities go to Resources C.

HIGH HISTAMINE

Whole families can have high histamine levels. 75% of these include high achievers, great athletes, CEO's, MDs, or scientists. 20%, however, may have hyperactivity, depression, aggressiveness, obsessive/compulsive behavior, and a racing brain. They may grow obsessive about sex, cry easily, have abnormal fears, and contemplate suicide.

DIRECTIONS

Check "yes" or "no" for each question below.

	YES	NO	
1.	____	____	Do you tend to sneeze in bright sunlight?
2.	____	____	Were you a shy and oversensitive teenager?
3.	____	____	Can you make tears and saliva easily and never have a dry mouth?
4.	____	____	Do you have a high sensitivity to pain?
5.	____	____	Do you get headaches regularly?
6.	____	____	Do you have seasonal allergies, such as hay fever? (75%)
7.	____	____	Do you need only five to seven hours of sleep each night?
8.	____	____	Are you a perfectionist or an obsessive, Type-A personality who feels driven?

SCORE YES ANSWERS _____

If you have any of the disorders listed in the beginning of this chapter and you scored "yes" to FOUR or more questions, you may benefit from laboratory testing of your histamine level.

© 2013 This questionnaire, originally developed by Carl Pfeiffer, PhD., has been updated by Suka Chapel-Horst, RN, PhD, in consultation with William J. Walsh, PhD.

For the location of recommended laboratory testing facilities go to Resources C.

LOW HISTAMINE

Histamine is a major brain neurotransmitter that causes incredible chaos when it rises to abnormal highs or falls dangerously low. If people have too *little* histamine, they may experience panic, anxiety, sleep disorders, bipolar symptoms, suicidal thoughts, psychosis, or schizophrenia.

MAJOR INDICATIONS

Check "yes" or "no" for each question below.

YES	NO	
____	____	Do you have slow sexual responsiveness or a low libido? (adults)
____	____	Do you have heavy growth of body hair? (adults)
____	____	Do you have a head full of grand plans but are easily frustrated?
____	____	Are you suspicious of people or do you feel paranoid?
____	____	Is your mouth usually dry? Do you have dry eyes?
____	____	Do you have a tendency to despair, or have bouts of crying?

SCORE YES ANSWERS _____

INDICATIONS THAT ARE OCCASIONALLY PRESENT

YES	NO	
____	____	Do you get canker sores?
____	____	Do you have tension headaches or seldom have headaches?

_____	_____	Have you ever heard voices inside your head?
_____	_____	Are you able to stand pain well?
_____	_____	Do you get few or no colds?
_____	_____	Do you need at least eight hours of sleep, and are you a slow riser in the morning?
_____	_____	Do you experience frequent irritability?

SCORE YES ANSWERS _____

If you have any of the disorders listed in the beginning of this chapter and you answered "yes" to **four** or more of the MAJOR INDICATIONS, you may benefit from laboratory testing of your histamine level. Ask your Health Care Provider to order laboratory testing of both your histamine and copper levels. Excess copper destroys histamine in the brain. This can cause violent behavior and depression, as well as paranoia.

Answering "yes" to **some** of the OCCASIONALLY PRESENT questions may be a further indication of low histamine and high copper levels.

© 2013 This questionnaire, originally developed by Carl Pfeiffer, PhD., has been updated by Suka Chapel-Horst, RN, PhD, in consultation with William J. Walsh, PhD.

For the location of recommended laboratory testing facilities go to Resources C.

TOTAL ACCUMULATED SCORES

You can place your scores from all the previous tests here for easy reference. As you move through your *recovery phase* you will find it helpful and encouraging to retake some of the tests and compare your later scores to the earlier ones.

TEST SCORES Date _____   REDO TEST SCORES   Date _____

_____ CARBOHYDRATE ADDICTION (Chapter 4)   _____

_____ CANDIDA (Chapter 5)   _____

_____ FOOD ALLERGIES (Chapter 6)   _____

_____ HYPOGLYCEMIA (Chapter 7)   _____

_____ HYPOTHYROIDISM (Chapter 8)   _____

_____ ADRENAL INSUFFICIENCY (Chapter 9)   _____

_____ ALCOHOL SCREENING (Chapter 10)   _____

_____ PYROLURIA (Chapter 11)   _____

_____ HIGH HISTAMINE (Chapter 12)   _____

_____ LOW HISTAMINE (Chapter 13)   _____

For recommended laboratory testing go to Appendix C - Resources.

PART TWO

Steps To Recovery

FIRST STEP TO RECOVERY

Now that you've done your testing to uncover any underlying conditions that need to be addressed (hopefully you've done that and followed through with the suggestions at the end of each test), you're ready to begin your *Recovery Phase*.

No matter what your current health condition is, there is one step that can improve your health immediately. Every organ and body system will benefit. It is the single, most important step you can ever take to regain optimal health. You probably already know what it is but are you doing it?

Prior to 1890 the U.S. sugar consumption was 20 pounds yearly per person. Today sugar consumption is 135 pounds yearly per person. In my high school class of 103 students, there was only one "fat" person. (We didn't even know the word "obesity".) Heart disease, cancer, and depression were rare. ADD/ADHD, learning disorders, childhood diabetes and depression were almost unknown. Addiction rates were far lower than today. Life expectancy was expanding (now it's declining). Today 37.5% of US Americans are obese and 68% are overweight. That means that today, a high school class of 103 has 68 overweight teens.

Do you find this as disturbing as I do? The good news is that there is a simple and doable solution for those who are willing to embrace it, but let's first look at the power of sugar to damage our lives.

The truth is that overconsumption of sugar is slow and progressive suicide.

Sugar/Corn Syrup Addiction is Responsible for:

Asthma	Hypertension
Arthritis	Depression
Diabetes	Heart disease
Obesity	Mood swings
Gall stones	Irritability
Cancer	**Personality changes**

Sugar/Corn Syrup Addiction in Children is Responsible For:

Obesity	Anxiety disorder
Addiction	**Criminal behaviors**
Depression	**Oppositional Defiant Disorder**
Type 1 Diabetes	

Hypoglycemia (low blood sugar due to an excess of insulin attempting to regulate sugar levels) is responsible for multiple symptoms and a majority of Americans are chronically hypoglycemic.

SOME SYMPTOMS OF HYPOGLYCEMIA (See Chapter 7 for a longer list.)

- ✓ nervousness
- ✓ irritability
- ✓ exhaustion
- ✓ hunger
- ✓ depression
- ✓ drowsiness
- ✓ insomnia

- ✓ mental confusion
- ✓ constant worrying
- ✓ internal trembling
- ✓ forgetfulness
- ✓ headaches
- ✓ negativity
- ✓ unprovoked anxieties

The single most important step to lowering blood pressure, normalizing blood sugar, reducing aches and pains, relieving depression and mood swings, eliminating irritability and angry outbursts, normalizing sleep patterns, decreasing behavioral problems, and improving relationships is to reduce sugar intake.

EXCESSIVE SUGAR IS POISON
Sugar is four times more addictive than cocaine

BREAKFAST CEREAL IS 75% SUGAR
"What are you giving your children for breakfast?"

We begin our first step to recovery by greatly reducing the intake of sugar in all its forms which include the *white* foods. Read ingredients on all food packages. Don't buy packaged foods if any form of sugar is first, second, or third on the ingredient list. Once you have achieved optimal health, *small* amounts of sugar won't be harmful.

Watch people in the grocery story putting white bread, chips, and sodas into their grocery cart. I guarantee that they will be overweight and/or have multiple emotional or physical health issues.

Sugar = Whites

Ice Cream

White flour pasta

White bread

White rice

White potatoes

White flour baked goods

List of Sugar Names

Agave nectar

Barbados Sugar

Barley malt

Beet sugar

Blackstrap molasses

Brown sugar

Buttered syrup

Corn syrup

Corn sweetener

Corn syrup solids

Crystalline fructose

Date sugar

Demerara Sugar

Dextrin

Dextran

Dextrose

Diastatic malt

Diatase

D-mannose

Evaporated cane juice

Ethyl maltol

Florida Crystals

Free Flowing

Fructose

Fruit juice

Fruit juice concentrate

Galactose

Glucose

Glucose solids

Golden sugar

Golden syrup

Granulated sugar

Grape sugar

Grape juice concentrate

HFCS

Cane crystals

Cane juice crystals

Cane sugar

Caramel

Carob syrup

Castor sugar

Confectioner's sugar

High-fructose corn Syrup

Honey

Icing sugar

Invert sugar

Lactose

Malt syrup

Maltodextrin

Maltose

Mannitol

Artificial Maple syrup

Molasses

Muscovado sugar

Organic raw sugar

Panocha

Powdered sugar

Raw sugar

Refiner's syrup

Rice Syrup

Sorbitol

Sorghum syrup

Splenda

Sucrose

Sugar

Syrup Syrup

Table sugar

Treacle

Turbinado sugar

Yellow sugar

The sugar industry is constantly coming up with new sugar names. Be on guard for new hidden sugars with insulin spiking ingredients. Some white breads are colored to look like whole grain.

THE THREE ROBBERS

It won't come as any surprise that there are three robbers who steal away our optimal health. They pretend to be wonderful, giving us the lift we want but they work in the hidden dark of our bodies to rob us of the very life we desire. Indeed, they steal our inner treasures, leaving us tired, irritable, frustrated, groggy, foggy and anxious.

You know who the three robbers are: junk food, sugar and excessive caffeine. They steal the quality and years of our lives while granting immediate and short-lived gratification.

Send them packing. You can cut the sugar and junk food out of your life immediately, just as you would slam the door on an unwanted intruder. Your best friends, the aminos (see Chapter 20) will easily give you the lift, or relief, you desire without any negative side effects.

Ah, the caffeine! It's best to usher this robber out more slowly. Reduce your intake over a two week period. A couple of cups in the morning isn't a problem. This is a guest that you can allow in for a *brief* daily visit, as long as there are *no* negative side effects (let down, anxiety, tension, etc.).

Even a *little* sugar won't harm you. But A LOT OF SUGAR will. If you are addicted to these robbers, you are aware of the negatives they are producing in your life. A "cuppa" coffee now and then, even one or two in the morning if you're *not* having any anxiety following it, is OK. Having a *very* occasional Dairy Queen, or burger with fries, is alright if there are NO negative side effects and you can easily say "no" to them AT ALL TIMES. But, if you *can't say no* and *can't stop* and *crave* caffeine, junk food, and sugar, you've got robbers, not guests.

This chapter is called *The First Step* for a reason. When you get control over just these three robbers your health will take such a jump forward you may find that's all you need to do. Even my own medical doctor said that if all his patients lowered their sugar intake, he would lose 70% of them as patients.

The benefits you may experience from reducing sugar intake include:

✓ Weight loss
✓ Lowered blood pressure
✓ Normalized blood sugar
✓ Reduction in aches and pains
✓ Decreased anxiety

✓ Relief of depression
✓ Improved sleep
✓ Decreased irritability
✓ Improved focus and concentration
✓ MUCH, MUCH MORE

Do you have to handle the robbers alone? No. Your bodyguards are the micronutrients you will be taking, along with healthy nutrition and exercise to get oxygen to your brain. But, even if you only send the robbers packing, and do nothing else, you will benefit. (Of course, after the robbers are gone, there is nothing left to eat but healthy food. Hmm.)

FIND IT. FIX IT. LIVE WELL.

*"Do you want a magic pill that will cover up the symptoms
or do you want to find the underlying cause and repair it?"*

Some people want the magic pill, the quick fix. They have suffered too long. They are tired. They believe that they have exhausted their options. Their disease labels have given them fear instead of hope, so they take their medications, often many medications. Never mind the side effects, the dangers. "Just give me relief." When they get some relief, they become afraid to get off the medications, even if they are also gaining weight, feel a bit "out of it", are lacking in energy, and so on. My heart goes out to them. I understand.

There is another option. It's one of hope and real recovery. Instead of disease labels, it offers a pathway to optimal health. Instead of painting over the rusty car, remove the rust and rebuild the car.

In case you bypassed the introduction, I'll repeat here that this book is a first step, an introduction to a subject that is far more complex than the simple strategies given here. Not all conditions can be relieved by these suggestions. Optimal health is the very best that is possible for *you*. You may need the guidance of an integrative health-care professional and if you do need it, please do get that help.

Meanwhile, you will benefit from what you learn in this book and you will definitely find your health improving if you follow the suggestions. Many of you will experience full recovery from your symptoms while others may need more intensive help but all of you will have a good head start to recovery.

When clients call me for a consultation, they know there is no such thing as a magic pill. They are ready for recovery. We begin a partnership to uncover the underlying cause of their symptoms and to develop a program leading to optimal health and wellness, based upon hope, not fear.

That process begins with some education about the biochemistry of the brain and body so that they can knowingly participate fully in the decision-making and follow-through necessary to achieve wellness.

So let's begin by learning about the brain's messengers, because they are the point where our recovery begins.

BRAIN'S MESSENGERS

The nervous system moves energy throughout the brain and spinal cord sending messages to every part of the body. Some nerves serve automatic functions like heart and lung activity while other nerves serve the conscious part of the brain which we can control. Nerves are not a continuous string. They're made up of independent cells that both receive and send messages through electrical impulses.

The messages, or electrical impulses, are carried from one neuron to another by chemical messengers called neurotransmitters. Over 100 neurotransmitters have been identified by scientists so far, and there are many more we are still learning about.

In the case of moodiness, depression, addictions, aches and pains, we'll focus on four of those neurotransmitters and their actions upon the brain.

FOUR BODYGUARDS

- DOPAMINE is the NATURAL ENERGIZER BUNNY
- SEROTONIN is NATURAL SUNSHINE
- GABA (gamma amino butyric acid) is NATURE'S CHILL-OUT TONIC
- ENDORPHINS are NATURE'S LOVE BUGS of COMFORT and PLEASURE

DOPAMINE – NATURAL ENERGIZER BUNNY

This neurotransmitter stimulates or excites us. It's called the "feel good" chemical. It governs our ability to pay attention and to experience excitement and pleasure. Some symptoms of a dopamine deficiency are:

- Depression
- Irritability
- Low energy
- Weight gain
- Sleep disturbances
- Distractibility
- Poor concentration
- Poor focus

- Poor memory recall
- Difficulty waking up in the morning
- Laziness
- Low motivation
- Lack of remorse
- Detachment
- Social withdrawal
- Suicidal thoughts

SEROTONIN – NATURAL SUNSHINE

This neurotransmitter is the relaxer. It lifts us from unpleasant emotions. It affects moods, sleep, appetite, and perception. It, along with GABA, moderates excessive dopamine levels and works to keep us in emotional balance.

Julia Ross, author of *The Mood Cure* and *The Diet Cure*, believes a serotonin deficiency may be affecting more than 80% of Americans. Eric Braverman, MD, author of *The Edge Effect*, believes that only 17% of the population produces enough of the "feel good" neurotransmitter. Some symptoms of a serotonin deficiency are:

- Depression
- Anxiety
- Panic attacks
- Irrational emotions
- Anger
- Irritability
- Impatience
- Phobias
- Negativity
- Low energy
- Lack of self esteem
- Lack of self confidence
- Poor concentration
- Eating disorders
- Premenstrual syndrome
- Inflexibility
- Decreased sex drive
- Guilt
- Violence
- Antisocial
- Behavior
- Suicidal thoughts

GABA - NATURE'S CHILL-OUT TONIC

This neurotransmitter (gamma amino butyric acid) acts as a sedative and helps to alleviate anxiety and worry. It works with serotonin to moderate excessive dopamine levels. GABA is the brain's natural valium. Some symptoms of a GABA deficiency are:

- Anxiety
- Panic attacks
- Nervousness
- Exhaustion
- Tension
- Sleeplessness
- Overwhelmed
- Pressured
- Overacting
- Seizures

ENDORPHINS – NATURE'S LOVE BUGS

These neurotransmitters are the brain's natural pain killers including both emotional and physical pain. They are 1000 times more powerful than heroin. People who are deficient in endorphins don't have the chemical ability to tolerate pain well. Women have greater deficiencies than men. Endorphins also gently stimulate the release of dopamine and the accompanying euphoria or good feelings that dopamine provides. Some symptoms of an endorphin deficiency are:

- Low pain tolerance
- Chronic pain (e.g. back aches, headaches)
- Very emotionally sensitive
- Depression

- Cry easily (e.g. from sentimental TV commercials)
- Find it hard to get through losses or grieving
- Difficulty experiencing pleasure
- Overly responsible or time urgent

REWARD DEFICIENCIES

When we have deficiencies in neurotransmitter levels, we experience what biochemist Kenneth Blum, PhD, calls a Reward Deficiency Syndrome. ("Syndrome" means a group of symptoms.) We don't get the natural rewards we hope for. We can't focus or concentrate as well as others. We don't get excited like other people do. We don't laugh as much. We aren't as happy. We're missing the rewards of life and we can't seem to do anything about it.

So, what causes neurotransmitter deficiencies? There are two kinds of reward deficiencies.

INHERITED GENETIC DEFICIENCIES

We can inherit these deficiencies from our parents. In this case, there will be a history of addictions, emotional or mental illness in the family. It may skip a generation but if it is inherited, it will be in the family somewhere. The inherited genetic coding is a protein recipe that determines the levels of neurotransmitters in the brain. With Reward Deficiency Syndrome, the neurotransmitter levels will be deficient from birth. Most individuals who are addicted to substances have this inherited deficiency and are drawn to the substance that supplies the missing reward in an attempt to self-medicate.

ACQUIRED DEFICIENCIES

Neurotransmitter deficiencies can be acquired during one's lifetime. In this case, a more rapid recovery may occur when the underlying imbalances are determined and rectified. Some of the sources of acquired neurotransmitter deficiencies are:

- Malnutrition
- Candida
- Food allergies
- GMO foods (genetically modified organisms)
- Chemical allergies
- Hormone imbalances
- Toxic metals
- Molds
- Intestinal disorders
- Alcohol / Drug *abuse*
- Chronic stress
- Trauma

Of course, we want to feel good. So, when we have chronic deficiencies, most of us look for ways to feel better and there are solutions that do make us feel better, at least for awhile. Let's take a look at how we may attempt to self-medicate.

SUBSTANCES USED TO PROVIDE THE MISSING REWARD

DOPAMINE DEFICIENCY

- Sugar
- Refined carbohydrates
- Caffeine
- Diet pills
- Tobacco
- Marijuana
- Alcohol
- Ritalin
- Adderall
- Cocaine
- Crack
- Amphetamines
- Methamphetamine

SEROTONIN DEFICIENCY

- Sugar
- Refined carbohydrates
- Junk food
- Marijuana
- Alcohol
- Remeron
- Wellbutrin

- Effexor
- Cymbalta
- Prozac
- Zoloft
- Paxil
- Celexa
- Lexapro

GABA DEFICIENCY

- Sugar
- Refined carbohydrates
- Junk food
- Marijuana
- Tobacco
- Alcohol
- Valium
- Librium
- Ativan

- Zanax
- Serax
- Klonipin
- Ambien
- Lunesta
- Restoril
- Prosom

ENDORPHIN DEFICIENCY

- Sugar
- Refined carbohydrates
- Junk food
- Marijuana
- Tobacco
- Alcohol
- Oxycontin
- Hydrocodone
- Vicodin
- Codeine

- Lortabs
- Fentanyl
- Darvocet
- Avinza
- Morphine
- Dilaudid
- Pallidone
- Heroin
- Methadone
- Suboxone

As you can see, when neurotransmitters are out of balance, too much or too little, the result is physical, emotional, and mental distress or illness. (Above-normal elevations of dopamine are involved with several mental and emotional disorders.) See Note

It's important to remember that if you are the driver of a vehicle that isn't performing properly (biochemically) *you* are not to blame for how you feel and how you sometimes react.

YOU ARE NOT A LABEL.
YOU ARE NOT A DISEASE.
DO NOT PUT YOURSELF DOWN!!!
THERE IS HOPE FOR RECOVERY.

The good news is that these neurotransmitters can be rebalanced. But understand, rebuilding and rebalancing neurotransmitter requires natural substances, the substances that they are made from, not synthetic molecules (pharmaceutical medications).

HOW DO WE REBALANCE BRAIN CHEMISTRY NATURALLY?

Protein is the indication of life because all living organisms are made of protein. Neurotransmitters are made of the components of protein which are amino acids. However, in order for amino acids to convert into specific neurotransmitters, vitamins, minerals, fatty acids, trace elements, and enzymes are required to assist in the metabolic process. We are what we eat. (*Babies are made from the mother's food, not from Prozac.*)

The process of metabolizing these substances is highly specialized. Co-factors, food supplements, are required in specific amounts at specific times in order to convert nutrients to brain and body chemicals. Skipping breakfast, gulping junk food for lunch, and eating a hefty dinner doesn't provide the right kind or amount of nutrients for maintaining balanced brain chemistry, much less repairing long standing existing imbalances. Some of the most common "foods" people eat and drink daily, and some medications, are further imbalancing brain chemistry, not repairing it.

The importance of just a single vitamin, for example, has far reaching effects on the whole body/mind process. In Chapter 21 I'll give you an example of just how powerful one vitamin alone can be. It's neither the most nor the least important vitamin, however, the example will serve to demonstrate just how important each and every nutrient is.

NOTE: In this book I am addressing only neurotransmitter *deficiencies* as related to moods, depression, and addictions. *Elevated* neurotransmitter and copper levels experienced by those with bipolar disorder and schizophrenia require the medical supervision of an integrative healthcare professional. Laboratory testing can provide a detailed analysis of the biochemical imbalances underlying these conditions and they can be successfully addressed with micronutrient therapy and nutrition. There is HOPE FOR RECOVERY without the side effects and dangers of pharmaceutical medications.

ABOUT MOODS AND DEPRESSION

- ✓ *"I'm so excited, I can hardly wait."*
- ✓ *"I know this is going to turn out badly. I can feel it in my bones."*
- ✓ *"I want to get out. I want to go somewhere and celebrate, anything."*
- ✓ *"I don't want to answer the phone today. Just leave me alone."*
- ✓ *"Bring it on. I can handle anything."*
- ✓ *"Everything is going wrong. What next?"*
- ✓ *"How do I feel? I feel great."*
- ✓ *"How do I feel? Not bad."*

Moods are either positive or negative. They can be responses to known situations or can occur for no identifiable reason at all. Moods can come and go. We can shift our moods if we choose to do so. Some people tend to be more negative and other people are more positive. When people change moods quickly or frequently, we call them "moody".

Moods affect our judgments, our reactions, and our decisions. They can be caused by outer circumstances and by inner health conditions. In this book we are addressing natural ways to have and hold positive moods. You have already learned how moods can be affected by neurotransmitter levels. If neurotransmitter levels are inadequate, we may have insomnia or anxiety, for example. This certainly affects our moods.

THE BLUES AND BLAHS

"I just feel down today. I don't have any energy. I want to curl up with a "fluff" book and read and don't talk to me because I want to be left alone."

"You go on to the dinner. Just tell them I have a cold (which I don't have). I don't feel like seeing anyone. My body feels like it wants to cry inside."

"I'm not really motivated or excited about this project. I know I started it but I don't feel the enthusiasm about it that I had earlier. I just want to get it over with and move on."

I'm sure you can come up with your own scenarios to describe the feelings of being "blue" or having the "blahs". It's natural to feel this way sometimes. Often you know the cause. Perhaps you didn't get enough sleep for a couple of nights in a row. Maybe you ate too much sugar and low carbohydrate foods recently. Maybe you are so overstressed or overwhelmed with circumstances or responsibilities in your life that you just "crashed". Maybe your mind has been going "full steam ahead" and you've been pushing yourself to the brink. Now you are in rebound. Your body is saying "slow down" and "let me catch up".

If this is happening all too frequently, you are probably in adrenal overload. You body is attempting to rebalance itself by slowing you down. As you read further in this book you will learn how to use the amino acids to keep you in balance when times are stressful. You will be able to read the signs and prevent most of the "blues" and "blahs" from occurring again. Acquiring good nutritional habits will help prevent these "downers" from sapping the life out of you. Your life will be naturally richer and more enjoyable, more of the time.

NORMAL DEPRESSION

It is healthy to be depressed when we have a loss or change that takes away family, friends, animals, places, jobs, or when a situation negatively changes how we view our self. Feeling depressed is a healthy and normal emotion because sadness, like all emotions, needs to be accepted and felt in order for it to be relieved. Stuffing negative emotions can lead to serious and chronic depression, as well as unexplained angry outbursts, weight gain, and decreased physical health.

When situationally caused depression is allowed to progress through its natural course, it will gradually dissipate and we will regain the ability to experience happiness and feel good again. The length of time it takes to readjust depends upon the severity of the loss or change.

During this time, we will have faster healing when we take advantage of the amino acid support, along with a healthy nutritional program. Often, during times of sadness and loss, we forget to eat. We may not even want to eat. That's a typical reaction. It's OK to eat less, as long as it continues to be balanced. The aminos will be a very good friend at this time.

SEASONAL AFFECTIVE DISORDER (SAD)

This seasonal depression is due to the lack of Vitamin D3. In North America most people are deficient in this vitamin. (See chapter 21.)

POST PARTUM DEPRESSION

Post-partum depression is often due to the failure of the normally high serum copper level that exists during gestation, to return to normal after the birth. Post-partum depression may be quickly relieved when the copper level is restored to normal. Months of depression are due to the failure of physicians to understand the underlying cause and repair it.

DEPRESSION

"I can still function. I do my job well at work. Nobody is complaining. I come home, fix dinner, spend time with the children, send them off to bed, and then I collapse. I just want to curl up in bed and hide. Nothing in my day was fun. I don't enjoy food.

I don't enjoy my children. I have no sexual desire for my husband and I avoid his sexual advances. I keep up a good front. No one seems to know that I'm just not "there." I've felt this way for awhile but I don't feel bad enough to see a doctor about it. I'll get over it. It's just a matter of time."

Maybe this woman would benefit from an antidepressant, temporarily. However, a better solution would be to find out what the underlying cause of her depression is. Because she hasn't mentioned any triggering event, I would suggest to her that she do some testing, find out what is going on biochemically, and repair it so that the depression would resolve naturally.

If she begins taking an antidepressant, she will add to her biochemical imbalances, become addicted to her medication, and feel bad about herself for having a medical diagnosis of an "emotional disorder". Furthermore, the underlying cause of her depression would continue to be unrecognized and unrepaired. She will either become dependent upon her medication or re-experience the depression, probably more deeply, if she stops the medication.

This is a typical scenario. Far too many men, women, *and* children are being medicated without testing for and repairing the underlying cause. It's just too easy to prescribe a pill and send the patient on their way.

CHRONIC DEPRESSION

Dr. William Walsh, PhD, a biochemist, began working with Carl Pfeiffer in 1978 to study clinical depression. He has more than 300,000 chemical analyses of blood and urine for 2,800 depressed persons. He discovered that this depressed population was biochemically different from the general population and has determined five depressive biotypes.

Each of these biotypes is caused by different biochemical imbalances and the restorative treatment differs with each. One biotype responds well to SSRI antidepressants while others do not. One biotype has a folate deficiency. Another biotype has excessive serum copper levels.

Another depressive biotype is due to pyroluria, a test you took earlier in this book. And another type of depression is caused by toxic overload.

Dr. Walsh is one of the world's best authorities on biochemical imbalances in schizophrenia, depression, autism, behavioral disorders, ADHD, and Alzheimer's disease.

His treatments include rebalancing the biochemistry with micronutrients, co-factors, nutrition, and with occasional, limited use of medications. Dr. Walsh trains physicians throughout the world. I recommend his recently published book *Nutrient Power-Heal Your Biochemistry and Heal Your Brain*.

Treating chronic depression is outside the scope of this book. For qualified medical help seek out integrative healthcare practitioners. You will find appropriate laboratory testing facilities listed in Appendix C.

BIPOLAR DISORDER

When individuals present with symptoms of depression that don't fall into a typical category, they tend to be lumped under the label of *bipolar disorder* especially if they have both apathetic and manic episodes. This is a shame. Labels don't tell the story. The symptoms do. No two people are alike. Many people have biochemical imbalances that can be corrected. Let's remove the labels and treat the underlying symptoms.

Dr. William Walsh theorizes that true bipolar disorder is not due to biochemical imbalances. He postulates that the problem may be more centered around the issue of physics and the electrical circuitry of the body. Certainly, science does not yet understand this disorder.

That said, I refer you to the book *A Promise of Hope* by Autumn Stringam available at www.TrueHope.com. (See Appendix D.) Many individuals with a diagnosis of bipolar disorder are having good success in recovery with a well researched nutritional product that can be ordered through this website, as well.

THIS BOOK

The purpose of this book is to inform people about this "other" world of health and healing "outside" the box of traditional, conservative medicine. The science and evidence-based studies for nutritional medicine are every bit as thorough and sound as those of traditional medicine. In truth, because there are no pharmaceutical gains to be made with nutritional medicine, the scientific evidence is unbiased and far more accurate.

Call it *orthomolecular* or *functional* or *integrative* medicine, it's the medicine Hippocrates was speaking of so long ago. I invite you to explore this expanding world of science and medicine.

This book is a reporting of the "tip of the iceberg". If you need more than this book can provide you, please read the books listed in Appendix D.

ANTIDEPRESSANTS – THE ON/OFF SWITCH

✓ *"Should I take an antidepressant?"*
✓ *"I've been on an antidepressant for a month and haven't noticed any change."*
✓ *"My antidepressant worked for about six months but it isn't working anymore."*
✓ *"When I tried getting off the antidepressant, my symptoms came back right away so I know I can never get off the medication."*
✓ *"My doctor says I have to stay on my antidepressant for at least six months, even though I don't want to take it anymore."*
✓ *"Will I ever be able to get off the antidepressants?"*
✓ *"When my medication dosage was increased, why did I became irritable, anxious, and restless?"*
✓ *"Can I just quit my antidepressant 'cold turkey'?"*
✓ *"Why do I have to take bigger and bigger doses of my medication?"*
✓ *"I'm frustrated with weight gain and lowered sexual drive, but I'm afraid to get off my antidepressant and go back to how I was feeling before."*
✓ *"Why do I have to take another antidepressant on top of the first one?"*
✓ *"Can I ever be well without the antidepressant?"*

These are just some of the questions and statements I hear from clients. People are confused. There is a growing awareness in the public about the side effects and dangers of antidepressant medications but many physicians prescribe them without adequately educating patients about how the medications work, about the side effects and dangers, and about how to stop taking them. Indeed, physicians are more apt to increase dosages instead of attempting to wean patients off the medications.

Although this chapter did not appear in the original version of this book, I've included it here due to the increasing number of calls I'm receiving as the result of my speaking to organizations and at conferences. If you are not taking an antidepressant, you can skip this chapter if you like, although having this information will give you the opportunity to inform others and help to prevent needless suffering.

WARNING
ANTIDEPRESSANTS ARE DANGEROUS AND ADDICTIVE DRUGS

✓ These drugs are frequently prescribed needlessly and indiscriminately.
✓ These drugs are usually prescribed without prior laboratory testing for cause.
✓ These drugs are often poorly monitored by the prescribing physician.
✓ Some of these drugs have been found to be no better than placebos in several trials.
✓ Patients using these drugs will become addicted to them.
✓ Patients will experience withdrawal symptoms when attempting to come off them.
✓ These drugs do not repair the underlying cause of depressive symptoms.
✓ These drugs can and do have mild to serious emotional and medical side effects.

Changes, up and down, in antidepressant dosages have resulted in violent behavior, violent suicide, and manslaughter.

ANTIDEPRESSANTS – WHAT DO THEY DO?

All antidepressants manipulate neurotransmitter levels. Depression is the result of low serotonin combined with either low or excessive dopamine, or excessive norepinephrine, which is made from dopamine. (Low dopamine leads to apathetic depression and the treatment is to increase the dopamine level.) Excess dopamine can lead from anxiety all the way to violent behaviors. Serotonin regulates dopamine levels. When serotonin is low, it can't modulate excessive dopamine levels. So the role of antidepressants is to regulate either serotonin or norepinephrine levels or both.

The first antidepressant usually prescribed for people is an SSRI (selective serotonin reuptake inhibiter) medication. These medications keep more of the existing serotonin available for use but do NOT increase the levels of serotonin. Over time, the existing serotonin becomes degraded and some is lost in the brain making less, not more, serotonin available for use as time goes on.

At first the increased availability of serotonin lifts the depression and reduces symptoms by either lowering excessive dopamine levels or simply by having more serotonin available to lift the depression. However, over time the serotonin is being depleted, and because no new serotonin is being made, it takes bigger and bigger doses of the SSRI to keep what serotonin is left in circulation. This may mean changing to another SSRI or adding a second one to the first antidepressant. In all cases, eventually, the serotonin reaches such a low level that there is little or no relief from the antidepressants.

The SNRI's act in the same manner by affecting the level of norepinephrine with the same kind of results. Other antidepressants *manipulate* the neurotransmitters in a different manner.

ANTIDEPRESSANTS DO NOT INCREASE SEROTONIN LEVELS

Antidepressants do not cure the underlying cause of the symptoms of depression. They create a remission of symptoms that will return when the medication is discontinued unless the underlying cause is removed.

SOME ANTIDEPRESSANTS BY NAME

- SSRI: Paxil, Zoloft, Prozac, Celexa, Lexapro, Luvox, Symbyax
- SNRI: Effexor, Cymbalta, Serzone
- OTHER: Wellbutrin, Remeron

ANTIDEPRESSANTS – HOW DO THEY WORK?

It usually takes about a month for the brain to adjust to an antidepressant. That's why people often don't feel any effects for several weeks after starting the medications. It then takes about six months for the brain to fully adjust. That's why coming off the medication before six months is premature for getting the full benefits.

From six months to a year after beginning the medication, adjustments may need to be made to continue to experience the desired effects.

ANTIDEPRESSANTS – HALF LIFE

Some antidepressants have a short half life. Others are long acting. A half life is the time it takes for half of the medication to clear the liver and be excreted from the body. Some antidepressants have a half life of five hours and others can be as long as six days. The shorter the half life, the more dangerous the drug is.

For example, Effexor has a five hour half life. If the patient forgets to take her medication on time, she will start to experience withdrawal symptoms and may not be aware that the symptoms are due to her failure to take the medication. She may think the medication isn't working or that the symptoms are due to something else. In fact, the drug is not available and she is really in withdrawal. Her symptoms are withdrawal symptoms that can be very uncomfortable and even dangerous.

On the other hand, Prozac has a half life of four to six days. A missed dose won't cause withdrawal symptoms and it is easier to taper off this medication.

ANTIDEPRESSANTS – CHANGE OF DOSAGE SERIOUS WARNING

**Whenever the dosage is changed, either up or down,
a change in moods and/or behavior can be expected (See Appendix A).**

The changes can be mild or as extreme as suicidal thoughts or violent behavior towards others. Any and every change in dosage, either up or down, MUST be closely monitored by the prescribing healthcare practitioner. Physicians should make set appointments to see their patient at the exact date the effects are due to begin. This date depends upon the half life of the drug.

Immediately contact your healthcare provider if any disturbing symptoms occur. These can be emotional reactions or medical emergencies. When people are taken to the emergency room or picked up by the police for behaviors that are not acceptable or safe, often the fact that the person has had a recent change in the dosage of their antidepressant medication is not reported. Many times, the medical people in the emergency room are unaware of the effects of medication changes. Sometimes brain scans and other expensive tests are performed when the simple and quick, almost immediate cure, is to reinstate the original dosage.

ANTIDEPRESSANTS – SUICIDE, VIOLENCE

When depressed people who are NOT on antidepressants are suicidal, they are seeking to escape feelings of guilt, self-loathing, despair, and hopelessness. Their suicidal acts are very rarely violent.

People who ARE taking antidepressants commit *violent* suicide due to an excess of dopamine which causes feelings of intense anxiety, pressure in the head, and feelings of exploding inside. They can experience heightened paranoia, irritability, and rage reactions from which they are compelled to escape. These same feelings can and do lead to manslaughter, as well.

These people will use weapons, knives, automobiles, throw themselves off buildings or bridges, even create suicide by police action.

CAREFULLY MONITOR ANY CHANGE IN DOSAGE – UP OR DOWN

Quickly call 911 if any serious withdrawal symptoms develop. Report the recent change in dosage and demand a return to the original dosage, or take the usual dosage if you have access to the medication.

ANTIDEPRESSANTS – MUST-HAVE REFERENCE

An excellent reference for understanding antidepressants, how to handle emergencies, and how to *safely* get off these medications is *The Antidepressant Solution* by Joseph Glenmullen, MD. This book is available at www.alibris.com and is a *must read* book.

If you are currently taking an antidepressant or are contemplating starting one, you should own and read this book for your safety. Not only will it assist you in preventing serious problems, but it will help you to know when and how to end your dependence on antidepressants. These medications should not be a life-long solution. When taken for good reason, they should be a short-term solution for stabilization, only.

You may have to be very assertive with health care providers who are poorly informed, but, if you have read this book, you will know how to get the right help when you need it.

ANTIDEPRESSANTS – SHOULD I TAKE THEM?

From the last chapters, you know:

1) There may be underlying causes that, when addressed, will alleviate your symptoms. Some of these conditions are reflected in the tests you did in the first part of this book.

First and foremost, thyroid deficiency, if present, must be addressed. You will want to address allergies, candida, hypoglycemia, and other underlying causes, if present. There may be hormonal issues that your healthcare practitioner will have to address. There can be intestinal and digestive deficiencies to address. Everything works together to complete the entire puzzle.

I suggest that you should not even consider taking an antidepressant until sufficient testing has been done to determine the underlying cause. The next step is to rectify the underlying cause. That done, depression and all the symptoms you are experiencing may be completely alleviated.

2) While testing for the underlying cause is going on, make sure your nutrition is healthy and appropriate (Chapters 22 and 23).

3) Test yourself for neurotransmitter deficiencies (Chapter 19) and begin taking the appropriate amino acids (Chapter 20) after first checking the *Precautions*. Once these procedures are undertaken, the need for antidepressants will often be gone.

ANTIDEPRESSANTS – HOW DO I GET OFF THEM?

If you have been on an antidepressant for a month or more, you MUST decrease the dosage a little at a time. Up to a month the brain has not yet adjusted to the change. That's why many people decide to quit. They haven't felt any different and think the drug isn't working. It is working but it takes time for the brain to adjust. If you have been on the drug less than a month, it is OK to stop it with your healthcare provider's supervision.

If you have been on the antidepressant one month or longer, you need to lower the dosage very carefully. The amount to decrease varies from person to person and drug to drug depending upon the half life of the drug. If you decrease your dosage by the appropriate amount once every four weeks, you should have only very mild withdrawal effects. (Withdrawal dosages are outlined in *The Antidepressant Solution.*)

ALL ANTIDEPRESSANTS ARE ADDICTIVE AND HAVE WITHDRAWAL SYMPTOMS

Introduced in the 1950's, the old tricyclic and heterocyclic antidepressants were routinely tapered off because of their known withdrawal effects. Many of these medications are no longer prescribed and some are no longer available. However, if you are taking one of these medications, know that they have withdrawal effects also. Withdrawal symptoms occur with MAO inhibitors, as well, so be warned.

ANTIDEPRESSANTS –WITHDRAWAL WARNING

Dr. Glenmullen calls it the *Catch-22* effect. When people decrease their dosage, they will have withdrawal effects. They may not have been warned that all antidepressants are addictive. So when they have the withdrawal symptoms, they think that the depressive symptoms they had *before* taking the medication are returning. They then think that they can't get off the medication because they will immediately have their old symptoms back. This is not true.

The underlying depression will not return immediately upon stopping the medication. It takes approximately four to six weeks for the brain to return to the prior condition. The symptoms the person is experiencing are actually *withdrawal symptoms.* They are temporary and unrelated to the original condition for which the drug was prescribed.

You will have to experience some withdrawal symptoms but if you carefully taper off according to safe guidelines only once every four weeks, you should be able to live with the withdrawal symptoms for the two to three days it takes for them to stop.

Most physicians are trained to prescribe, not to decrease medications. Your physician may not know how to safely lower your dosage. Before telling your physician that you want to stop taking your medication, *please* read *The Antidepressant Solution.* You will have the information to educate your physician. You will know what *should* be done, if your physician does not. Take the book with you and stick to your knowledge. You would be amazed at how uninformed most physicians are about stopping a medication.

Your physician should set appointments to see you *in person* to evaluate your withdrawal symptoms *as they are happening.* This book will provide you with both the emotional and medical symptoms to expect and how to evaluate them. It will help you to safely decrease your medications, even if your physician is less than helpful.

The *Catch-22* is that when people notify their physicians that they are having symptoms, most doctors think that the original problems are returning. (You now know better.) Their solution is to *raise* the dosage to keep you from the old depressive symptoms. They are wrong. You are not returning to the old symptoms. You are in *withdrawal.*

If you are in doubt, remember that physicians are taught about these medications by pharmaceutical reps who are parroting the pharmaceutical line. They do not train doctors to lower dosages. They train them to increase dosages.

ANTIDEPRESSANTS and AMINO ACIDS TOGETHER

"I'm currently on an antidepressant but I'm going to get off it. Can I take the amino acids at the same time? What about the other supplements and the nutritional program?"

First, find any underlying cause. Your testing in the earlier chapters should begin that process. You may need to get some laboratory testing, as well. Secondly, your health will automatically improve when you reduce your sugar and low carbohydrate intake, as well as improve your nutritional habits, including *eating breakfast.*

Thirdly, begin taking the *Power Foods*, your food supplements (Chapter 22).

Fourth, after answering the questions in the Mood Meter (Chapter 19) you can begin taking the amino acids (Chapter 20). However, they will not have the same effect as long as you are on your antidepressant. As the antidepressant dosage decreases, the amino acid effects will begin to kick in more and more. You will have to trial the dosages as directed to learn what works best for you. Follow the amino acid guidelines carefully.

Taking the amino acids should help to reduce any withdrawal effects you may have as you decrease your antidepressant dosages. As always, immediately stop any amino that gives you a negative response. You can trial it again at a later date.

ANTIDEPRESSANTS AND YOU

I cannot express enough how dangerous these drugs are. They are as addictive as benzodiazepines, opiates, and alcohol. They are NOT the benign medications doctors want you to believe. I hope you will inform your family and friends about what you have read in this chapter. You already know more about these drugs than many professionals in your medical community.

MOOD METER

Now let's find out which, if any, of your neurotransmitters (NTs) you may be deficient in. You may be deficient in more than one and that is common because they work together. (We are looking for deficiencies, not excesses.)

DIRECTIONS

1) In the **first column**, put a number from **zero** (no symptoms) to **ten** next to each symptom you have, with **one being slightly felt or hardly ever felt** and **ten being strongly felt or felt all the time**.
2) The second column provides you with a space to recheck how you are doing in the future and compare that number with your original numbers.
3) In the **third column**, **check** those substances that you **use**, or **have used**, to **reduce** the symptoms in column one.

LOW DOPAMINE – Energizer Bunny NT

Deficiency Symptoms	Redo Date	Substances Used
_____ apathetic depression	_____	_____ caffeine
_____ lack of energy	_____	_____ cocaine
_____ lack of drive	_____	_____ methamphetamine
_____ lack of focus, concentration	_____	_____ tobacco
_____ ADD	_____	_____ Wellbutrin
_____ crave substances for energy or focus	_____	_____ Ritalin
		_____ Adderall
		_____ marijuana
		_____ milk chocolate
		_____ sweets

LOW SEROTONIN – Sunshine NT

<u>Deficiency Symptoms</u>	<u>Redo Date</u>	<u>Substances Used</u>
_____ negativity, depression	_____	_____ sweets
_____ winter blues	_____	_____ starch
_____ worry, anxiety	_____	_____ tobacco
_____ low self-esteem	_____	_____ milk chocolate
_____ hyperactivity	_____	_____ Ecstasy
_____ obsessive thoughts or behaviors	_____	_____ marijuana
_____ perfectionist, controlling	_____	_____ alcohol
_____ irritability, rage (e.g. PMS)	_____	_____ Prozac
_____ panic attacks, phobias (fear of heights, snakes, small spaces, etc.)	_____	_____ Zoloft _____ Effexor _____ Lexapro
_____ fibromyalgia, TMJ, migraines	_____	_____
_____ afternoon or evening craving substances	_____	_____
_____ insomnia, disturbed sleep	_____	_____
_____ night owl, hard to get to sleep	_____	_____ Trazadone

LOW GABA – Nature's Chill Out NT

Deficiency Symptoms	Redo Date	Substances Used
_____ stiff, tense, or painful muscles	_____	_____ marijuana
_____ stressed/burned out	_____	_____ alcohol
_____ unable to relax, loosen up, get to sleep	_____	_____ Xanax _____ Ativan
_____ often feel overwhelmed	_____	_____ tobacco
_____ craving substances for stress relief	_____	_____ sweets/starch

LOW ENDORPHINS – Natural Comfort, Pleasure, and Love Bugs NT

Deficiency Symptoms	Redo Date	Substances Used
_____ very sensitive to emotional/ physical pain	_____	_____ starch _____ milk chocolate
_____ cry or tear up easily	_____	_____ marijuana
_____ history of chronic pain	_____	_____ alcohol
_____ love and crave comfort, pleasure, reward	_____	_____ Vicoden _____ heroin
_____ numbness from substances / behaviors		_____ caffeine
_____ excessive behaviors (e.g. exercise, porn, self-harm)		_____ tobacco

LOW BLOOD SUGAR - Hypoglycemia

Deficiency Symptoms	Redo Date	Substances Used
_____ irritable, shaky, stressed, especially if you go long periods between meals	_____ _____	_____ sweets _____ starches _____ alcohol
_____ cravings for sugar, starch or alcohol		_____

[Additional symptoms of hypoglycemia are nervousness, irritability, exhaustion, rapid pulse, depression, drowsiness, insomnia, mental confusion, constant worrying, internal trembling, forgetfulness, headaches, and unprovoked anxieties. All of these symptoms can be treated naturally by correcting the imbalanced brain chemistry.] Insert by Dr. Suka

If you have **several** scores of **8 to 10** in any of these categories, you are **probably low** in that neurotransmitter. **Reread** the lists of deficiency symptoms in the last chapter for additional clues.

[This test and information is reprinted with permission from Julia Ross, MA, Director of Recovery Systems, Mills Valley, CA, author of *Mood Cure* and *Diet Cure*.]

The solution is quite simple. You'll recall that neurotransmitters are made up of amino acids. So, in order to increase your neurotransmitter levels, you simply take the appropriate aminos to get relief from your symptoms. If you are deficient in a neurotransmitter, by taking the appropriate amino acid, you will begin to feel relief in five to fifteen minutes. Really!

Over several weeks or months of this stimulation, the biochemistry usually begins to "catch on", naturally increasing neurotransmitter production. However, the brain will always need sufficient amounts of amino acids to "feed" the process and food alone won't be enough. Additionally, as we age, neurotransmitter production alters. We, then, simply add the aminos as needed in order to maintain optimal health.

NOTE: Amino acids, taken *without* the co-factors that assist in metabolism, will not be sufficient to build or maintain healthy neurotransmitter levels. See Chapter 22, *Power Foods,* to learn more about these important micro-nutrients.

IMPORTANT: Before going further, read AMINO ACIDS PRECAUTIONS and DO NOT TAKE any amino acids that are contra-indicated.

AMINO ACID PRECAUTIONS

Please consult a <u>knowledgeable</u> healthcare practitioner before taking ANY amino acids if ANY of the following statements apply to you.

- You tend to react to supplements, foods or medications with unusual or uncomfortable symptoms.
- You have a serious physical illness, particularly cancer.
- You have severe liver or kidney problems (e.g. Lupis).
- You have an ulcer (amino acids are slightly acidic). [This does not apply if you take all amino acids under the tongue and do not swallow them.] Insert by Dr. Suka.
- You are pregnant or nursing (a complete amino blend is usually acceptable, but not individual aminos.)
- You have schizophrenia or other mental illness.
- You have phenylketonuria (PKU).
- You are taking any medications for mood problems, particularly MAO inhibitors or more than one SSRI/SNRI.

Please check off and avoid or be cautious about trying the supplements indicated on the right if you have:

(DL-Phenylalanine = DLPA)

High blood pressure	L-Tyrosine or D-Phenylalanine	DLPA
Very low blood pressure	GABA	
Migraine headaches	L-Tyrosine or D-Phenylalanine	DLPA
Bipolar spectrum tendencies	L-Tyrosine or D-Phenylalanine	DLPA
Bipolar spectrum tendencies*	L-Glutamine	
Severe Depression	Melatonin	
Asthma	L-Tryptophan & 5-HTP	Melatonin
Overactive thyroid or Hashimoto's	L-Tyrosine or L-Phenylalanine	DLPA
Excessively high cortisol output	5-HTP only	
Carcinoid tumor	L-Tryptophan & 5-HTP	
Melanoma	L-Tyrosine or D-Phenylalanine	DLPA
Lymphatic cancer	L-Glutamine	

* In approximately 50% of bipolar cases, L-Glutamine can trigger mania. *Note:* L-Glutamine can sometimes relieve bi-polar depression without triggering mania. (SAM-E, St. John's Wort, bright therapeutic lamps, and too much fish or flax oil may also trigger mania.)

Even if your health care provider agrees that you can try amino acids
(or any other nutrients), if you experience discomfort
of any kind after taking them, stop taking them immediately.

Name_____Date_____

© Julia Ross, author of *The Mood Cure* (Penguin 2004) and *The Diet Cure* (Penguin 2012)
This information is reprinted with permission of Julia Ross, MA, author of The Diet Cure and The Mood Cure.

AMINO ACID REPAIR

Amino acids are natural proteins, the building blocks of all life. We eat and drink them every day without a second thought. Excess aminos that our body can't use, are flushed from our system. (Alcohol flushes aminos out before they can be metabolized.) If our neurotransmitter levels are normal, we don't need amino acid supplements. However...

**If neurotransmitter levels are deficient, amino acids
must be present in order to restore neurotransmitter levels to normal.**

If you take an amino acid that you don't need, you may have a slight temporary negative reaction. If that occurs, discontinue taking that specific amino acid. Any negative reactions you may have are quickly resolved and are not serious, as long as you are following the Precautions in Chapter 19. (See General Instructions below.)

I am naturally high in Dopamine, the Energizer Bunny neurotransmitter. When I take Tyrosine, the dopamine precursor, I quickly get a slight head ache in the temple and I feel a little "off kilter" or dazed. So, I avoid taking that amino because my brain is not low in it.

Amino acids are precursors to the formation of neurotransmitters and specific aminos follow pathways to creating specific neurotransmitters.

NEUROTRANSMITTER PATHWAYS

AMINO ACIDS lead to the formation of NEUROTRANSMITTERS

➤ <u>L-Tyrosine leads to the formation of Dopamine, then to norepineprhine and epinephrine.</u>

➤ <u>L-Tryptophan leads to 5HTP which leads to the formation of Seratonin.</u>

➤ <u>GABA is an amino acid that leads to the neurotransmitter GABA.</u>

➤ <u>D-Phenylalanine (DPA) leads to DL-Phenylalanine (DLPA) which leads to the formation of Endorphins.</u>

➤ <u>DL-Phenylalanine (DLPA) also mildly increases Dopamine.</u>

➤ <u>L-Glutamine leads to the formation of GABA.</u>

SOME SPECIFIC AMINO ACID GUIDELINES

- SEROTONIN and DOPAMINE are opposites. Taking L-Tryptophan or 5-HTP (for Serotonin) and L-Tyrosine (for Dopamine) **together** will **cancel** each other out. As you will see in the protocol, we want the lift of Dopamine from morning to mid-afternoon and the relaxing effect of Serotonin from mid-afternoon through the evening.

- Because DL-PHENYLALANINE (DLPA) (for Endorphins) also increases Dopamine, take it only in the morning and up to mid-afternoon. For *physical* pain relief *after* mid-afternoon, take D-PHENYLALANINE (DPA).

- SEROTONIN leads to the creation of MELATONIN, the sleep aid. When taking Melatonin by itself fails to induce sleep, it's usually because the Serotonin level is too low. When insomnia is a problem, take TRYPTOPHAN instead of 5HTP. When there is adequate Serotonin, Melatonin will automatically start to develop as daylight fades. To induce sleep, two hours before going to bed, turn lights down low, reduce sounds such as the TV volume, and do things that don't require concentration. This will increase the amount of Melatonin that is being produced in preparation for a good night's sleep. If insomnia continues, add GABA in the afternoon and evening, as well.

- GABA assists Serotonin in regulating Dopamine levels. It can be taken anytime, as needed and in combination with any other amino acids to calm down, chill out, reduce anxiety, and relax. It's also helpful in reducing PTSD symptoms. If you have breathing problems after taking 500 mg of GABA, immediately discontinue it.

- L-GLUTAMINE is taken to relieve the symptoms of low blood sugar and whenever you are craving sugar, sweets, and alcohol. This amino does NOT need a trail. It's safe to take it as needed.

These guidelines are an introduction to the power of amino acids which can provide wonderful relief for many of your symptoms. If you discover something that works well for you, continue to take it without worry and enjoy the benefits. Of course, there is no single magic pill.

In order for the aminos to restore neurotransmitter deficiencies, the body's complex biochemistry requires the addition of the co-factors you will learn about in Chapter 22 as well as some other amino acids, not discussed here, that may also be necessary for improving your health.

If you want to learn more go to Appendix D for additional reading that can guide you further and answer more of your questions.

AMINO ACID PRECAUTIONS

Carefully read the precautions if you have not already done so. DO NOT take any designated amino acids that are contraindicated.

HOW TO BEGIN YOUR AMINO ACID TRIALS

We haven't talked about the co-factors that are needed to metabolize the aminos and we haven't covered any nutritional plans yet, however, you can go ahead and start trialing your amino acids now. To begin the trials,

1. Don't drink any caffeine on the day you will be doing the trials.
2. If you are currently taking any medications, trial the aminos in mid-afternoon so they will not be so affected by your medications.

GENERAL INSTRUCTIONS (For adults only.)

1. Before starting to take the aminos, **purchase** Vitamin C powder. You will use it if you have a negative reaction. If you don't have a negative reaction, you can still use the powder as a supplement (See Chapter 22, *Power Foods.*) It won't waste.

2. You can **swallow** the entire capsules if desired. However, the aminos will go to work more quickly if you take them on an empty stomach either one half hour before meals, two hours after meals, or in between meals. They are less effective if taken with meals.

3. You will get the **fastest effect** if you open the capsule and drop the powder **under your tongue**. Let the amino dissolve without taking water. It will go to the brain bypassing the stomach and digestive system for quicker relief. Toss the capsule. This is the **recommended** method.

4. **To begin,** you will **first trial your dosage, one amino at a time.** Start with the lowest dose, one capsule. Place the amino powder under your tongue, wait five to fifteen minutes and notice the effect. If you need more effect, you can take a second amino and wait another five to fifteen minutes to see the effect. Go up to the largest dosage only if needed. Once you have trialed the aminos and know what dosage works best for you, in the future, you can take that entire amount all at once. **Do not take more** than is needed to get the effect. **Do not trial more than one amino acid at a time.**

GENERAL INSTRUCTIONS (For children.)

Consider *age* and *sensitivity*. Trial the aminos in the same manner as with adults.

1. START with a low trial dose.
   a. Infants and sensitives: pinch
   b. Under age 13: ½ dose
   c. Over age 13: full dose

2. STOP:
   a. With any adverse reaction
   b. When they are no longer needed

NEGATIVE REACTION

1. If you get a **negative reaction, immediately stop taking the amino.** If you take too much of an amino, you can get the very reaction you are trying to alleviate. Do not continue to take any amino that gives you a negative or reverse reaction. This is why you trial the amino and the dosage in the beginning. **NEVER take more than one capsule at a time until you have completed the trials.** It may be too much for you.

2. For quick (minutes) relief add 1000 mg of powdered Vitamin C to 4 ounces of water, stir and drink. Aminos naturally leave the body in one to four hours.

WHICH AMINOS SHOULD I TAKE? (For Adults only – See Children Instructions above)

Go back to your Mood Meter results in Chapter 19. If you had several 8's, 9's or 10's with any neurotransmitter, you will most likely benefit from the amino that stimulates that particular neurotransmitter.

KEY: NT – Neurotransmitter, AM – on arising, B – breakfast, MM – mid morning, L – lunch, MA – mid afternoon, D – dinner, BT – bed time

DOPAMINE – ENERGIZER BUNNY NT (Excitatory)

Benefits: Alertness, Drive, Mental focus, Enthusiasm

L-Tyrosine
500-2000 mg AM, MM, MA by 3:00 PM
or
DL-Phenylalanine (DLPA)
500-2000 mg AM, MM, MA by 3:00 pm
Stimulates endorphins and dopamine but is less potent than taking L-Tyrosine directly.

SEROTONIN – SUNSHINE NT (Antidepressant)

Benefits: Positive outlook, Flexibility, Feel good, Sense of humor

L-Tryptophan
500-2000 mg 2-4 times between MA and evening by 8 PM
or
5-HTP (Faster acting than L-Tryptophan)
50-200 mg 2-4 times between MA and evening by 10 PM if sleep is a problem.

The choice between taking L-Trytophan versus 5-HTP depends on why you are taking it. If the need is physical, use L-Tryptophan. If the need is emotional take 5-HTP which is closer to the end result and works faster.

Use in the evening if symptoms persist or if sleep is a problem.
May use if you wake up in the night. May add GABA 100-500 mg if needed.

Melatonin for eight hours of deep restful sleep. Take 3 mg for sleep at ideal bedtime *if* the above does not work alone, or for shift workers.

REMINDER
SERATONIN and DOPAMINE are OPPOSITES.

*Taking L-Tyrosine or DLPA **and** Tryptophan or 5HTP together will cancel each other out.*

GABA – CHILL OUT NT (Tranquilizer)

Benefits: Calmness, Relaxation, Stress tolerance, Reduces anxiety

GABA
100-500 mg anytime as needed. May take at bedtime to assist sleep.

and/or
Inositol Powder – 1000 mg in water 1 to 4 times daily as needed for anxiety/panic. This Vitamin B is tasteless. Prevents anxiety build-up and panic attacks.

and/or
L-Taurine
500 mg up to three times daily for calming and stabilizing. Building block for all neurotramsmitters. Works with all neurotransmitters.

and/or
L-Theanine
100 mg up to three times daily. Supports serotonin levels. Reduces anxiety. Found in green tea.

ENDORPHINS – COMFORT, PLEASURE, LOVE BUGS NT (Pain Relief)
Benefits: Physical and emotional pain relief

D-Phenylalanine (DPA)
500-1500 mg AM, MM, MA 2-4 times a day
or

DL-Phenylalanine (DLPA)
500-2000 mg AM, MM, MA 2-4 times a day by 3:00 pm
If the need is physical take D-Phenylalanine (DPA). If the need is emotional take DL-Phenylalanine (DLPA).

If become nervous or agitated after taking DLPA, decrease the dosage or take D-Phenylalanine (DPA) instead.

LOW BLOOD SUGAR (Hypoglycemia)
Benefits: Fuel source for all brain cells. Sense of stability and groundedness, blood sugar balance. REDUCES CRAVINGS FOR SWEETS AND ALCOHOL.

L-Glutamine
500-1500 mg AM, MM, MA In addition, take as needed for cravings.

Add Chromium 200-300 mcg at each of 3 meals for chronic hypoglycemia
9:10

Amino acids can't work by themselves. In order for them to be transformed into neurotransmitters, other vitamins and minerals (cofactors) must also be present. These include the masterful Vitamin B's, Vitamins C and D3, calcium, magnesium, essential fatty acids, and others. That's why healthy nutrition, coupled with the Power Foods (supplements), is necessary for everything to fall into place.

The next chapter tells the story of just one vitamin. If one vitamin has all these effects, you can easily imagine how powerful and necessary each and every vitamin is. I've selected Vitamin D3 for this chapter because the research is relatively new and many people are still unaware of the importance of natural vitamin D3. (Avoid synthetic D2.)

MANAGING YOUR SUPPLEMENTS TIP

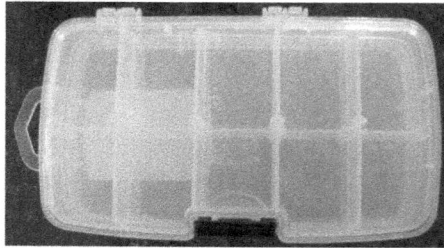

You can purchase small fishing tackle boxes that will easily hold several days' worth of supplements and aminos. These boxes are easy to pack for traveling. I package our supplements in several boxes to last for a month at a time. For those times when we are out all day, we just slip our supplements into small baggies and off we go.

PURCHASING YOUR AMINO ACIDS AND SUPPLEMENT CO-FACTORS

You can purchase these supplements at health food stores, food co-ops, or online. To order high quality amino acids, go to www.BrainworksRecovery.com.

SUNSHINE MAKES ME HAPPY

"Sunshine on my shoulders makes me happy."
John Denver

How right John Denver was! So right, that I've devoted a whole chapter to the wonders of sunshine, and more specifically, to Vitamin D3.

To begin with, Vitamin D is not really a vitamin at all. It's a powerful steroid hormone. However, we will stick with the name it's popularly known by. (Just thought you might find that interesting.)

The information in this chapter is excerpted, with permission of the author, from the book *Vitamin D3* authored by Paul Stitt, MS, CNS, one of the biochemists who pioneered the research studying the effects of vitamin D3 deficiency.[1] This is NOT the most important vitamin but it serves to point out the power of just one single co-factor (a necessary supplement for the metabolism of the amino acids.)

Vitamin D3 plays a HUGE part in maintaining optimal health. Paul Stitt called it the *Fountain of Youth*. Deficiencies lead to all of the following conditions.

VITAMIN D DEFICIENCY LEADS TO:

- Arthritis
- Alzheimer's disease
- Rheumatoid Arthritis
- Autoimmune diseases
- Cancers
- Depression
- Diabetes
- Emphysema
- Chronic Bronchitis

- Fibromyalgia
- Gout
- Kidney disease
- Lupis
- Parkinson's disease
- Premenstrual Syndrome
- Pregnancy
- Schizophrenia
- Tuberculosis

DEPRESSION

Vitamin D3 helps to produce serotonin – the SUNSHINE neurotransmitter. A deficiency can contribute to depression. *Alternatively, increase Vitamin D3 levels and both moods and positive attitudes will be elevated, sometimes within as little as fifteen minutes.*

John Cannell, MD, a California psychiatrist, states that about 90% of his patients in a mental health center are Vitamin D3 deficient. 90%!! When placed on a Vitamin D3 regimen, mood disorders are improved.[2]

Seasonal Affective Disorder (SAD) is directly associated with lack of sunlight and a Vitamin D3 deficiency. Almost everyone feels less energized, physically and emotionally, during a series of gray days. Night-shift and indoor workers suffer, as well, from an occupational affective disorder.

High stress may increase the need for Vitamin D3, magnesium and calcium. People with Parkinson's and Alzheimer's diseases have lower levels of Vitamin D3. Studies show definite improvement when they receive Vitamin D3 and a high-fiber, highly nutritional diet.

People will experience a rapid improvement in both mood and energy in just five days of Vitamin D3 supplementation. Because of climate, latitude, and lifestyle, year-round Vitamin D3 supplementation is recommended.

ARTHRITIS

Arthritis affects 40% of Americans and 50% worldwide. It's more common than heart disease or cancer and dates back thousands of years. An estimated 50 million adults in the United States reported being told by a doctor that they have some form of arthritis, rheumatoid arthritis, gout, lupus, or fibromyalgia. In 2007–2009, 50% of adults 65 years or older reported an arthritis diagnosis.[3]

The **real cause of arthritis is a lack of Vitamin D3** from the sun or in the diet from early age. When understood, this condition can easily be prevented by insuring that children maintain an adequate level of Vitamin D3. For those of us who are older, we can immediately improve our Vitamin D3 level with supplementation.

Some people may have increased pain and inflammation due to eating members of the nightshade family. These include:

- Potatoes
- Peppers
- Eggplant
- Huckleberry

- Tomatoes
- Ground Cherries
- Garden Huckleberry

To find out if these foods are increasing your pain, stop eating them for one month and see if the pain is reduced. When reintroducing them, if there is no increase in pain, you don't have to eliminate them from your diet. If there is an increase in inflammation or pain, you can then make an informed decision about what you will and won't eat.

I used to drink a small can of V8 juice every day. I found that it did, indeed, cause me discomfort and had to give it up.

SIX TIPS TO TREAT AND MANAGE ARTHRITIS

1. Increase Vitamin D3 consumption to a minimum of 5,000 IU daily. You may go as high as 20,000 IU for three months before backing off to 5,000 IU daily to maintain appropriate levels of vitamin D3.
2. Use cayenne pepper to control pain and increase circulation. (See Chapter 22.)
3. Avoid *all* dairy for two weeks, then test to see if the pain is worse after dairy products are reintroduced.
4. Eat fruits, vegetables, protein (preferably animal protein – chicken, turkey, fowl, fish, occasional grass-fed beef, lamb) healthy fat, and whole grains daily.
5. Drink lots of water.
6. Exercise and stretch daily as much as possible without doing harm.

Glucosamine and chondroitin can aid in joint restoration. Fruits, vegetables, meat, fish and eggs contain methyl-sulfonylmethane (MSM) which helps to relieve pain and inflammation in joints and muscles. In addition, it boosts blood supply, lessens muscle spasms and softens scar tissue. It's also helpful to massage affected areas and use topical preparations for pain.

CANCER

Vitamin D3 deficiency weakens white blood cells that fight infections and kill cells that can become cancerous increasing the risk for colon, mammary, prostate and ovarian cancer by 30% to 40%. Vitamin D3 is essential to the form and function of every cell in the body. Evidently, when some cells don't get enough Vitamin D3, they go wild and attack each other. The cells start growing uncontrollably, forming tumors and destroying their host.

One study done at Harvard University found that Vitamin D3 almost tripled the five year survival rate of patients with lung cancer. *Other studies show that patients who avoided milk had 35% less risk of having either breast or prostate cancer.*

DIABETES

Cow's milk produces an antibody that destroys the part of the body that produces insulin. *Cow's milk products drastically increase the risk of diabetes.* Diabetics will flourish on a healthy diet of natural foods and foods high in fiber. Avoid all dairy products, and foods made of bleached white flour, hydrogenated fats and corn syrups. In addition take:

- 200 mg chromium daily (Consult your healthcare provider for higher dosages.)
- ½ teaspoon cinnamon daily
- 5,000 IU Vitamin D3 daily

EMPHYSEMA & CHRONIC BRONCHITIS

Vitamin D3 helps to prevent these conditions. Studies show that people with low levels of Vitamin D3 have more breathing problems than former smokers who were getting adequate levels of vitamin D3.

WEAK MUSCLES

Vitamin D3 deficiencies lead to weak muscles and frail bones which lead to falls and fractures. Most nursing home patients have low levels of Vitamin D3.

Deficiencies in Vitamin D3 increase the risk for heart disease because heart muscle cells become weak and unable to pump blood efficiently.

OSTEOPOROSIS

Vitamin D3 deficiencies lead to osteoporosis and humped-back shoulders in the aged. Researchers state that falls and fractures could be cut in half in 3-6 months if people consumed enough Vitamin D3.

OSTEOPOROSIS QUIZ

1. Do you have chronic pain every week?
2. Do you use any type of pain killer on a weekly or daily basis?
3. Did your mother lose height as she aged?
4. Are your muscles weaker now than they were 10 years ago?
5. Have you suffered a fracture?
6. Do you suffer from PMS?

If you answered "yes" to any of these questions, you should have your blood checked for 25 Hydroxy D3 levels. The least expensive and most accurate Vitamin D3 test can be obtained by going to www.vitamindcouncil.com. You don't need a prescription.

Let's look at a common myth. *"Milk makes strong bones and teeth."* Studies have shown that milk intake has no effect on later bone strength. Most people can't absorb Vitamin D3 from milk due to curd formation. In fact, excess calcium blocks Vitamin D3 from being activated in the body. Calcium becomes toxic at high levels and blocks absorption of iron, zinc, magnesium, etc. (Veterinarians use high levels of ionized calcium to euthanize cats!)

Soda "pops" due to phosphate which leeches calcium from the bones – visualize teens and sodas during the very time their bones are developing. Cow's milk is also a major source of phosphate. Processed meats and soft cheeses that melt easily have added phosphate, as well as high salt levels that also leech calcium from bones.

Estrogen therapy is not recommended for women with osteoporosis. Excess steroids can cause osteoporosis and fractures.

Another common myth is, *"Exercise to build bones."* Surprisingly, exercise without an appropriate Vitamin D3 level does not build bones. Healthy bone growth requires Vitamin D3, calcium, magnesium, and omega 3 fatty acids.

A maximum of 1,000 mg calcium daily is sufficient to build healthy bones, if coupled with 5,000 IU Vitamin D3, daily.

PREGNANCY

Early in pregnancy, a deficiency in Vitamin D3 can increase the risk of type-I diabetes in the child. The deficiency can also cause slow brain development, which may lead to a child being born with a lower IQ.

SKIN PIGMENTATION

African American's skin pigmentation protects those who normally reside in sunny tropical climates, however, the darker the skin, the more exposure from the sun it needs to make Vitamin D3. African Americans absorb only 2% to 50% as much of the Ultra-Violet rays from the sun as Caucasians.

People with darker skin experience twice as much chronic pain, arthritis, bone fractures, ovarian, uterine and breast cancer, colon cancer, prostate cancer, heart disease, diabetes and many other chronic maladies. People of color need about 5,000 IU of Vitamin D3 daily for optimal health.

Lactating women of color need 5,000 IU of Vitamin D3 daily in order to help prevent soft, painful bones in the baby and diabetes. Vitamin D3 will improve learning ability in the child.

Immigrant women who practice orthodox religions by keeping their bodies and faces completely covered have severe Vitamin D3 deficiencies and need Vitamin D3 supplementation.

PRESCRIPTION DRUGS

Many drugs increase the need for Vitamin D3. Anticonvulsant drugs induce osteoporosis and many bone problems. Dr. Drezner from the University of Wisconsin recommends that people on anti-epileptic drugs should automatically be given at least 2,000 IU of Vitamin D3 per day plus 600 mg of calcium. ("We think these dosages are too low." Stitt) *Doses of 15,000 IU per day may be needed for those with muscle-bone pain.* She does not recommend the use of Fosamax™ for such patients. Paul Stitt also recommends the addition of foods that are fortified with magnesium, folic acid, B-6 and B-12.

Vitamin D3 is not patentable and is very inexpensive to produce. Drug companies are invested in *relieving* pain, not *preventing* it or *repairing* the underlying condition. Most drugs create side effects that require additional drugs to mask the side effects.

Vitamin D3 gives only beneficial effects.

TOXICITY

Experience has shown that Vitamin D3 dosages as high as 40,000 IU daily are safe. Toxic levels have occurred when Cod Liver Oil is taken in excess and from injections. Also, Vitamin D2, a synthetic form, can be toxic. Vitamin D3 is a safe natural form.

A million units a day of Vitamin D3 is probably toxic. Only two people have been harmed (not killed) by an overdose by ingesting over a million IU daily, according to the scientific literature.[4] 40,000 IU is on the high side, but is not dangerous for most people.

People who spend lots of time outdoors have been getting over 10,000 IU a day with no problems.

OPTIMUM LEVELS

One can achieve optimum levels of Vitamin D3 by exposing the arms and head for 20-30 minutes four days a week in noonday sun in warm climates. More time is required in higher latitudes. Seasonal and climate changes, as well as lifestyle, make this almost impossible for most of us.

Alternatively, a full tablespoon of cod liver oil taken daily helps but doesn't taste very good or one can get enough Vitamin D3 by eating 5 pounds of liver and 50 eggs daily. Supplements are quicker, easier, and effective.

It may take up to 10,000 IU of Vitamin D3 daily to build one's body up to a healthy Vitamin D3 level. After five months at these levels, one can usually maintain a healthy Vitamin D3 level with 5,000 IU daily, year round.

In addition, maintain a diet high in fruits and vegetables, to ensure adequate intakes for magnesium, potassium, Vitamin D3, Vitamin K and other nutrients.

Egg yolks and sardines contain Vitamin D3 but eating fatty fish doesn't work very well because Vitamin D3 is in the fat of the fish which most people won't eat. An exception is salmon, a good source of the vitamin. And you may have to eliminate dairy products.

An optimal 25-D blood concentration for most people is 80 to 100 nmol/1. Therefore, have your blood checked for 25 Hydroxy D3 and try to maintain a level of at least 100 nmol/1 (about 5,000 IU daily).[5]

1 *Vitamin D*, Paul A. Stitt, MS,CNS,M Natural Press, 2006

2 *Vitamin D*, Paul A. Stitt, MS,CNS,M Natural Press, 2006, p 103

3 Center for Disease Control and Prevention, *MMWR* 2010;59(39);1261-1265.
   [Data Source: 2007–2009 NHIS]

4 *Vitamin D*, Paul A. Stitt, MS,CNS,M Natural Press, 2006, p 113

5 *Vitamin D*, Paul A. Stitt, MS,CNS,M Natural Press, 2006, p. 114

POWER FOODS – CO-FACTORS

Vitamins, minerals, essential fatty acids, enzymes and trace minerals are the co-factors that are necessary to metabolize the amino acids. In the past, people didn't think much about supplements because the food they ate was nutritious and supported all their needs. Not so today. Even organic foods are subject to depleted soils, acid rain, airborne chemicals, and polluted water. Animals are raised on grasses that no longer have essential nutrients. Then they are fed corn (genetically modified and lacking nutrients) to fatten them up.

Late last July I drove past fields where they were beginning to pick tomatoes. There was not a single ripe red one anywhere on the vines. Since the nutrients develop only as the fruit or vegetable ripens on the vine, these green beauties had no nutritional value. In addition, the fields have not been allowed to lie fallow, nor have the crops been rotated. (Bacteria in the soil, that feeds the plants, multiply only when fields are fallow, or with crop rotation.) Looking pretty, red, and ripe, doesn't mean vine ripened.

So, in order to get well-rounded nutrition, optimal health *requires* supplementation. In the last chapter, you learned how precious Vitamin D3 is for all-around health. To further understand just how important individual vitamins are, let's consider the Vitamin B's.

Vitamin B's do not all have numbers. They are really just a collection of supplements grouped under the Vitamin B heading.

If there are deficiencies in Vitamin B's, the following can result:

DEFICIENCY	RESULT
B1 Thiamine	Memory loss, central-nervous system damage, numbness and tingling in the arms and legs, mental confusion, nervousness, headache, poor concentration
B3 Niacin	Depression, fatigue, apprehension, headache, hyperactivity, insomnia
B5 Pantothenic Acid	Depression, irritability, tension, dizziness, moody, quarrelsome
B6 Pyridoxine	Anxiety, nervousness, depression, convulsions, extreme nervous exhaustion, poor dream recall
B7 Biotin	Depression, lethargy, hallucinations, numbness/tingling of extremities (Deficiencies are rare)

B9 Folic Acid	Agitation, moodiness, headaches, depression, fatigue, decreased sex drive, confusion,
B12 Cobalamin	Lack of concentration, impulsive, angry, decreased memory, depression
Choline	Poor memory, gastric ulcers, high blood pressure, cardiac symptoms, kidney/liver impairment
Inositol	Irritability, mood swings, panic attacks, obsessive-compulsive behavior, arteriosclerosis, constipation, hair loss, high blood cholesterol, skin eruptions

Enriched wheat and refined white flour bread, buns, doughnuts, etc. have over 90% of the B vitamins removed. Alcohol flushes Vitamin B's and amino acids out of the body. Pyroluria, if present, also removes both the Vitamin B's and zinc from the body through the urine.

The Vitamin B's MUST be present, in the proper amounts, in order for amino acids to be transformed into the neurotransmitters and we cannot get enough of this vitamin from food sources to restore neurotransmitter deficiencies.

SUPPLEMENT FORMULAS

The following food supplements are suggested to encourage optimal health for most people. These may vary from person to person. Of course, you should choose the supplements that will meet your individual needs

The **Basic Formula** is suggested for most people. The **Optional Nutrients** are suggested if you have special health needs that require more than the Basic Formula offers. Add the **Optional Nutrients** to meet your individual needs.

DO NOT SACRIFICE QUALITY FOR COST

Poorly compounded supplements are immediately flushed from the body with no effect except to deplete your pocketbook.

SUGGESTED BASIC DAILY FORMULA

- ✓ Vitamin/Mineral Formula appropriate for your age and gender
- ✓ Vitamin B6 50 mg two to three times daily. Vitamin B is converted into P-5-P.
    Scot/Irish people don't absorb B6 very well.
    For better bioavailability, take P-5-P.
- ✓ Vitamin B12 1000 mcg 1 daily
- ✓ Vitamin C 2000-3000 mg with bioflavonoids. Sustained Release in divided, daily doses minimum
- ✓ Vitamin D3 5000 IU minimum. For SAD (Seasonal Affective Disorder), low energy, or sadness take up to 20,000 IU daily)
- ✓ Vitamin E 400 IU 1 daily
- ✓ Calcium / Magnesium (2/1 ratio) to equal 1000 mg Calcium daily for females (Can take in divided doses)

✓ Magnesium 300 mg daily
✓ Omega 3 3000 mg daily (Take in divided doses) or Ground Flax Seed
           (Fish oil, or Krill oil is easier to digest than Flax Seed Oil)
✓ Garlic Kyolic 2 daily or one onion or garlic bud daily
✓ Greens Powder if not eating enough vegetables
✓ Antioxidant formula daily

SUGGESTED OPTIONAL NUTRIENTS FOR SPECIFIC NEEDS Take as needed.

Arthritis	Chondroitin & Glucosamine (Comes from shell fish)
Cold Prevention	Echinacea Take for cycles of 8 weeks on and 1 week off in the winter.)
	Vitamin C - At the onset of a cold take 500 mg every hour for four hours.
Elevated Cholesterol	Red Yeast Rice plus CoQ-10 (Yeast destroys some CoQ-10 so it must be replaced regardless of your age)
Heart/Circulatory Disease	Cayenne (25% cayenne) One to two daily from Cayenne Company (See below) May increase "heat %" as able to tolerate plus CoQ-10 100 mg One daily.
Heart/Liver	Turmeric 500 mg twice daily
Ulcers	Cayenne (25% cayenne) One to two daily.
Hypoglycemia/Diabetes	Chromium 200 mcg daily. (Consult health care provider if taking insulin. Taking this nutrient may result in a reduction of insulin dosage.)
Over 50	CoQ-10 60 mg One daily
Yeast Infections	Acidophilus, Bifidophilus, and other probiotics
Anti-Aging	DHEA 5-25 mg (Get lab test first and monitor)

NOTE: When purchasing these supplements check for any ingredients that you may be allergic to, such as: wheat, gluten, soy, milk, eggs, fish, peanut oil, yeast, sugars, colors, preservatives, etc.

RECOMMENDED SOURCES FOR HIGH QUALITY SUPPLEMENTS

Anova Health 864-408-8320 Use code: DRSUKA5
www.BrainworksRecovery.com 417-380-3254
Life Extension: www.lef.org 1-800-678-8989
Bronson Vitamins: www.bronsonvitamins.com 1-800-235-3200
Cayenne Company: www.cayennecompany.com 1-800-229-3663

Disclaimer:
This information is not a substitute for medical advice from your healthcare practitioner.

EAT RIGHT FOR LIFE

Probably one of the most important books ever written on the subject of nutrition was *Nutrition and Physical Degeneration* by Weston A. Price, DDS. First published in 1939, republished many times and most lately in 2009, this book is a classic of research, and fascinating reading. (See www.westonaprice.org for more information.) Dr. Price, a dentist and his wife, spent many years visiting the native and aboriginal peoples in every part of the world. He measured and photographed the teeth and jaws of these people while keeping a journal of the foods they ate, their general health, and lifestyle.

These native people had no health diseases, healed quickly from wounds, and had perfect teeth and jaws. They had no jails, no need for police, and lived happy and congenial community lives. There was no obesity, no diabetes, heart disease, cancer, arthritis, or any other of today's common diseases including emotional and mental disorders. Yet, when they were exposed to missionaries and traders who gave them white flour, white sugar, jams, refined vegetable oils and canned goods, signs of degeneration quickly became evident. Dental caries, deformed jaw structures, crooked teeth, arthritis and a low immunity to tuberculosis became rampant amongst them. If their children returned to their grandparent's original way of eating before age fourteen, they had none of these deformities or diseases proving that the changes were not genetic, but were due to the changes in nutrition.

Regardless of where these people lived, whether by the sea or inland, in warm or cold climates, anywhere in the world, they had an instinctive ability to eat the foods that would maintain their health. Most importantly, their diets were high in animal protein and natural fats. It made no difference whether the protein and fats came from land animals or fish. They ate an abundance of it.

POP AND MOM FOODS –Protein and Fat

I call protein the POP food and fats the MOM food. We need POP and MOM. POP, or protein, provides us with the amino acids that create our neurotransmitters. MOM, or fats, make up approximately 70% of the brain and are necessary for life. Fats help nutrient absorption, nerve transmission, and maintain cell membrane integrity.

Did you know that we don't get fat (overweight) from eating fat? It's sugar and refined flour that makes us fat. *Also, a low fat diet can increase anger and hostility.*

What protein should we eat? Kosher meats, a small amount of red meat if desired, lamb, chicken, turkey and fish, along with plant protein, lentils, and nuts are excellent. *Avoid processed meats.* Because red meat is a storehouse for toxins and hormones, eat only grass fed animal meat. Eggs are an excellent source of protein, as well as dairy products *if* you are not dairy allergic. Vegetarians need to really "beef up" (sorry) their protein from whatever sources that are acceptable to them. No aboriginal tribe was vegetarian.

Healthy fats include butter, yes, real butter. It's wonderful for cooking because it can cook at a high temperature without creating free radicals (molecules that steal away the good nutrients). Coconut oils are also good for cooking. Extra virgin, cold-pressed olive oil is great for salads but not for cooking. Healthy fats are extra virgin olive oil, flax seed oil and fish oil. Fats from plant sources are nuts, seeds, avocados, and coconuts. Eat and enjoy.

FOOD PLAN DIRECTIONS

The following lists are foods you can eat to your heart's content. What was your score for Carbohydrate Addiction (Chapter 4)?

1. **Not positive** for a carbohydrate addiction? Use the **Optimal Health Food Plan.**
2. **Positive** for a carbohydrate addiction? Follow the **Low Carb Food Plan** for at least four weeks before switching to the Optimal Health Food Plan.

OPTIMAL HEALTH FOOD PLAN

If you are not addicted to carbohydrates, eat these foods and enjoy.

BEVERAGES

Apricot juice	Pineapple juice
Carrot juice	Raspberry juice
Clear broth	Sauerkraut juice
Herb teas	Tangerine juice
Grapefruit	Tomato
Herb teas	V-8 juice (not with arthritis)
Lemon juice	
Lime juice	
Loganberry juice	
Milk (Limited – See Allergies)	**(Dilute all fruit juices,**
Orange juice	**2 parts spring water to 1 part juice)**

WHOLE GRAINS
Barley
Buckwheat
Millet
Oatmeal
Rice (brown or wild)
Whole wheat

CHEESES
Cottage cheese
Cream cheese
Gouda, goat, or sheep cheese

Do not use processed cheese, cheese spreads, or squeeze-bottle cheese.

FRUIT (fresh)
Apples
Apricots
Avocado
Banana (limit to 1 daily)
Blueberries
Cantaloupe
Casaba melon
Cherries
Coconut (fresh)
Fruit salad (without grapes)
Grapefruit
Grapes (eat sparingly – high in fructose)
Honeydew melon

Lemon
Lime
Muskmelon
Oranges
Peaches
Pears
Pineapple
Plums
Raspberries
Rhubarb (no sugar added)
Strawberries
Tangerines
Watermelon

VEGETABLES (fresh)
Artichokes (globe or French)
Asparagus
Beans (green or wax)
Beets
Broccoli
Cabbage
Cauliflower
Celery
Cucumbers
Edamame beans
Lettuce
Mushrooms
Olives
Onions (green or raw)
Parsley

Peas (green or edible pod)
Peppers
Pickles (dill or sour)
Pimentos
Potatoes
Radishes
Rutabaga
Sauerkraut
Soybeans
Spinach
Squash (Hubbard or winter)
Tomatoes
Water chestnuts
Zucchini

SPROUTS
Alfalfa

Bean

PROTEIN

Chicken	Fish
Turkey	Meat (unprocessed) (limit red meat)
Wild game	Veal
Eggs	Lamb
	Shellfish

FATS

Butter	Extra virgin cold-pressed Olive oil
Coconut Oil	Avocado

SALT (half potassium/half sodium)
Morton's Lite Salt

RAW NUTS and **SEEDS**

Almonds	Pumpkin seeds
Brazil nuts	Sesame seeds
Peanuts	Sunflower seeds
Pecans	Walnuts

LOW CARB FOOD PLAN

If you are addicted to carbohydrates, eat only these foods for four weeks before changing to the Optimal Health Food Plan. Restrict carbohydrates to 50 to 75 grams daily. Dr. Atkins Gram Counter will be helpful with this.

ANY PROTEINS including:

Beef (unprocessed) (limit red meat)	Veal
Chicken	Lamb
Eggs	Fish
Turkey	Wild game

RAW NUTS and SEEDS

Almonds	Pumpkin seeds
Brazil nuts	Sesame seeds
Peanuts	Sunflower seeds
Pecans	Walnuts

VEGETABLES (fresh)

Avocado

Asparagus

Beans (string or wax)

Bean sprouts

Beets

Beet greens

Cabbage

Carrots

Cauliflower

Edamame beans

Eggplant

Kale

Okra

Onions (green or raw)

Peas

Pumpkin

Sauerkraut

Scallions

Spaghetti squash

Spinach

Summer squash

Swiss chard

Tomatoes

Turnips

Water chestnuts

Zucchini

SAFE FATS

Avocado

Butter

Cream Cheese

Olives

Mayonnaise (no sugar)

Extra virgin cold-pressed Olive oil

Yogurt-plain

Kefir

Buttermilk

Cottage cheese

Coconut oil

GRAINS

Wasa bread

Soy flour

Crispbread

FRUIT (fresh)   (High in carbs)

Melons

Berries

Grapefruit

FRUIT JUICES

Water them down to ¼ fruit juice and ¾   water

GREEN LEAFY LETTUCE and salad
fixings, such as:

Cucumbers

Radishes

Peppers

Herbs

Sprouts

Mushrooms

Olives

Jicama

Food plans are adapted from Seven Weeks to Sobriety by Joan Mathews-Larson, PhD

A WORD (or two) ABOUT GMO'S & BGH

Genetically Modified Organisms (GMO'S) are foods that have had a modified gene inserted into their natural genetic code. Created by Monsanto (the same company that provided chemicals for Agent Orange), these genes are implanted into **corn, soy, sugar beets, cottonseed** and other foods, to create a resistance to their product, Round Up®, and other herbicides.

When bugs eat the corn, their bellies explode. Gruesome, but there is more. These modified genes are transferred to cattle and then to human intestines where they continue to multiply and destroy the healthy bacteria in human intestines, creating a "leaky gut syndrome". This allows poisons to enter the blood stream while preventing healthy nutrients from moving into the blood stream.

Some of the symptoms linked to the ingestion of GMO modified foods are:

- Asthma
- Autism
- Cancer
- Infertility
- Decreased Immune System

- Leaky Gut
- Organ Damage
- Spontaneous Abortions
- Tissue Damage

BGH, or Bovine Growth Hormone, is given to cows to increase their milk production and is linked to an increased cancer risk.

JUST SAY "NO" TO GMO AND BGH

Be aware that genetically modified corn and sugar beets form most of the sweetening in all processed foods. Soy isn't safe, either, being genetically modified, as well. (See Appendix A for more disturbing information about soy.)

BASIC TIPS FOR OPTIMAL HEALTH

- AMINO ACID ADDICT: Become one.
- EAT three meals daily. Meals don't have to be big, just balanced with plenty of protein and vegetables.
- EAT BREAKFAST. Skipping breakfast is one of the major causes of obesity and alcohol relapse!
- EAT SLOWLY: Put silverware down between bites.
- PORTIONS: A portion is the size of your palm. Use small plates.
- SNACKS: Eat high protein, high fat snacks between every meal.
- POOP: Healthy poop floats. Check it out.
- URINE: Should be straw color or yellow if taking lots of Vitamin B's.
- SLEEP: Get seven to nine hours sleep every night.
- WALK or EXERCISE daily.
- PLAY, have FUN, LAUGH, Don't take things so seriously.
- HUG, KISS, AND LOVE A LOT.

- EXPECT GOODNESS and BLESSINGS to come to you all the time.
- BE GRATEFUL for all the good in your life and all the good that is coming into your life.
- BE HAPPY. It's more fun than not being happy. It really is your choice.

BLOOD TYPES

Dr. D'Adamo, author of the best-selling books, *Eat Right for Your Type* and *Live Right for Your Type,* presents a picture of our genetic heritage - the story line of our life. According to D'Adamo, even though we are living in the 21st century, we share a common bond with our ancestors. The genetic information that resulted in their particular characteristics has been passed on to us.

Why are some people plagued by poor health while others seem to live healthy, vital lives even late in life? Does blood type influence personality? A single drop of blood contains a biochemical make-up as unique as our fingerprints. Our blood type is a key to unlocking the secrets to our biochemical individuality. Foods and supplements contain lectins that interact with our cells depending on our blood type. This explains why some nutrients which are beneficial to one blood type, may be harmful to the cells of another.

You may find this information helpful to understanding how you are unique from others and why we are not all the same. Dr. D'Adamo's books are widely available if you want to pursue this further.

WATER, WATER, WATER

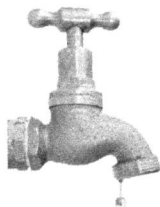

I've saved this for last because I want to make a BIG SPLASH of it. Water makes up 70% to 75% of our body. The nervous system, and all body systems, require enough water to function properly. Water removes toxins and waste from the body.

If we are not drinking enough water, our bodies become stressed and we will have multiple unwanted symptoms. Water in other drinks such as coffee or tea, does not count.

> Drink six to eight 8-ounce glasses of water every day *without fail.*
> Begin your day with one to two glasses upon arising.

CANDIDA AND ALLERGY REPAIR

Now that you've taken the Candida and Allergy tests you already have an idea of whether you are allergic to any foods or if you may have Candida. Let's deal with Candida first.

CANDIDA SYMPTOMS

- ✓ Depression
- ✓ Disoriented, spacey, light-headed
- ✓ Poor memory
- ✓ Difficulty concentrating
- ✓ Difficulty making decisions
- ✓ Bloating, distension, or gas
- ✓ Abdominal pain
- ✓ Loss of sexual interest or ability
- ✓ Vaginal burning, itching, or discharge
- ✓ Premenstrual tension or cramps
- ✓ Cold hands or feet or physical chilliness
- ✓ Pain or swelling in joints
- ✓ Chronic eczema, rashes, or itching (anal, under breasts)
- ✓ Body odor or bad breath not relieved by washing/brushing
- ✓ Chronic sore throat, laryngitis, cough, or tender glands
- ✓ Urinary frequency, burning, or urgency
- ✓ Pain or tightness in chest, wheezing, or shortness of breath
- ✓ Recurrent ear infections, fluid in ears
- ✓ Chronic sinus infections
- ✓ Have a sensitivity to mold
- ✓ Severe athlete's foot, nail or skin fungus, ringworm, or other chronic fungus
- ✓ Treated for internal parasites
- ✓ Crave or consume lots of sweets
- ✓ Crave or consume lots of starches such as pasta or bread
- ✓ Crave or consume lots of alcoholic beverages
- ✓ Food sensitivity or intolerance
- ✓ Persistent yeast infections
- ✓ Prostatitis, vaginitis, or other reproductive problems
- ✓ Frequently exposed to high-mold environments

Causitive Factors: Antibiotics and other drugs
- ✓ Taken tetracycline or other antibiotics for one month or longer
- ✓ Frequent short courses or other broad-spectrum antibiotics
- ✓ Taken prednisone or other cortisone-type drugs for one month or more
- ✓ Taken birth control pills for more than a year

If your test results indicate that you have Candida, follow the LOW CARB FOOD PLAN. You will be eliminating the sugars and starches that feed the Candida. Remain on this food plan for at least a month. Of course, you now know that reintroducing sugars into your food plan is a call for Candida to redevelop.

If the Candida persists while you are on this food plan, consult with your health care provider. Diflucan is a prescription drug that can be very helpful in speeding up your recovery. There are many good medications, some of which do work better than natural sources. Using medications with good judgment, and as minimally as possible, is wise. Homeopathy treatment can be very effective, as well.

ALLERGIES

Allergies can affect your digestive system, skin, respiratory system, muscular system, and more. The most severe allergic reaction is anaphylaxis, which affects many body systems and can be fatal.

The most common allergies are to wheat and dairy products. Allergies to milk and milk products can create severe behavioral and even criminal behaviors. The book *Food and Behavior* by Barbara Reed Stitt, PhD, is an eye-opener. As a Probation Officer, she worked with thousands of adults and school children. When they changed their diets, and removed the offending foods, their criminal behaviors stopped entirely and they became well-adjusted law-abiding citizens. Consider the impact this has on raising children who are difficult to manage. (Her book is available on our web site www.BrainworksRecovery.com.)

IF YOUR ALLERGY TEST WAS POSITIVE

Ask yourself some questions. "Can I easily give up this food?" "Am I reluctant to give it up?" "Do I eat it every day?" "Does it give me pleasure to eat it?" If you eat something every day, even several times a day, and don't want to give it up, you are most likely allergic to it. You may not be aware that the symptoms you are experiencing, such as arthritic or muscular pains, runny nose, rashes, depression, irritability and dozens of other symptoms are the result of an allergic reaction to this food that you so dearly love. ("Dearly loving it" is a clue!)

ELIMINATION DIET

The most effective method for determining if you are allergic to a food is the Home Testing Elimination Diet. This method is even more accurate than any blood or skin test. Here's how to do it.

Day 1 to 5 – Elimination

Stop consuming all the foods you have decided to test. For cravings, take your aminos according to your needs. (Become an Amino Acid Addict.) If you are allergic to any of the foods you are testing, you should start feeling better by day five.

Day 5 – The Challenge

1. Notice if any of your bothersome symptoms have gone away and make a written note of it.
2. On DAY FIVE eat a regular serving of ONE TEST FOOD ONLY for breakfast and again at lunch. Eat nothing else besides that product (an all dairy meal or wheat-only meal, for example).
3. Write down how you feel. Also note your oral temperature, any food cravings, your mood, energy, digestion, respiratory symptoms, bowel function, appetite, skin changes, headaches, sleep patterns and any and all information that your body tells you. You may have a very strong reaction, such as a migraine if you're prone to them. If you get only a little tired, bloated, or headachy after your challenge meals, don't ignore it. If you gain weight or start craving foods again, don't be surprised. It's very helpful to have someone with you when you test your food to observe reactions that you may not be aware of.
4. If you are testing grains for a gluten allergy, test wheat first as it contains the most gluten.
5. Do not eat any more of the food or food group for the next three days.
6. After waiting 72 hours, you can test another food group, milk for instance.
7. Don't eat any foods you have tested until you have finished testing all of the foods you have stopped.
8. Take DLPA or DPA to manage your side effects. (Chapter 20.)
9. If you have a negative reaction, you'll know what food or food group to avoid. If you accidentally eat the food and have a reaction, take two tablets of Alka Seltzer Gold to get rid of it quickly.

HELPFUL HINTS

1. Keep a detailed food-mood log to monitor your reactions
2. Reintroduce only one food group at a time.
3. Wait two full days before testing another food.
4. Be aware of ALL adverse reactions, no matter how small.
5. Women should test after their period and before PMS.

Delayed reactions, up to 48 hours, can occur so continue to monitor your reactions and write them down, no matter how small or unusual they may appear.

Some people have more severe intestinal problems which can take several months before the intestines can heal. If this testing is not sufficient, I refer you to *The Diet Cure* by Julia Ross, MA, for more detailed guidelines.

ALLERGY PROGRAM FOOD PLAN

Using this food plan, which automatically **eliminates** both **wheat** and **dairy** products, will make it easier to plan your meals. You can eat heartedly of any and all of these foods.

BEVERAGES

Apricot juice
Carrot juice
Clear broth
Herb teas
Lemon juice
Lime juice
Loganberry juice
Orange juice

Pineapple juice
Raspberry juice
Sauerkraut juice
Tangerine juice
V-8 juice (not with arthritis)

(Dilute all fruit juices, 2 parts spring water to 1 part juice)

FRUIT (fresh)

Apples
Apricots
Avocado
Blueberries
Cantaloupe
Casaba melon
Cherries
Coconut (fresh)
Fruit salad (without grapes)
Grapefruit
Honeydew melon
Lemon

Lime
Muskmelon
Oranges
Peaches
Pears
Pineapple
Plums
Raspberries
Rhubarb (no sugar added)
Strawberries
Tangerines
Watermelon

NUTS and SEEDS

Almonds
Brazil nuts
Peanuts
Pecans
Pumpkin seeds

Sesame seeds
Sunflower seeds
Walnuts

PROTEIN

Chicken and other fowl
Eggs
Fish

Meat (unprocessed) (limit red meat)
Shellfish

VEGETABLES (fresh)

Artichokes (globe or French)
Asparagus
Beans (green or wax)
Beets
Broccoli
Cabbage
Cauliflower
Celery
Cucumbers
Lettuce
Mushrooms
Olives
Onions (green or raw)
Parsley
Peas (green or edible pod)
Peppers
Pickles (dill or sour)
Pimentos
Radishes
Rutabaga
Sauerkraut
Soybeans
Spinach
Squash (Hubbard or winter)
Tomatoes
Water chestnuts
Zucchini

SPROUTS

Alfalfa
Bean

WHOLE GRAINS

Quinoa
Amaranth
Oats
Rice (brown or wild)

FATS

Extra virgin cold-pressed Olive oil
Coconut oil
Avocado

Food plan is adapted from Seven Weeks to Sobriety by Joan Mathews-Larson, PhD

WHAT'S THE FUTURE FOR THE ALLERGY PRODUCING FOODS YOU LOVE?

Remain free of the offending foods for six months. Then, one at a time, you can reintroduce them. Eat the offending food no more than once every four to five days. If you have several offending foods, alternate them so that you are eating only one of them a day.

As you begin to feel like a new person, you will agree that the effort was well worth it.

BEYOND NUTRIENT THERAPY

Identifying the underlying cause of less than optimal health and initiating appropriate nutrient therapy and healthy nutrition are the most important first steps to optimal health. As brain chemistry begins to correct, improvements in one's emotional and mental states seem to occur almost magically.

That said, we don't have to make the journey to optimal health by ourselves. There are many resources that can speed and enhance our recovery. Indeed, some of these resources may be *required* in order to release internal stressors and harmful habits. Let's look at a few.

FLEXIBILITY and EXERCISE - A MUST TO REGAIN OPTIMAL HEALTH

A daily stretching routine is *strongly recommended.* It takes only a few minutes with no equipment, special clothing or space requirements. You will feel so much better afterwards and your body and spirit will benefit beyond measure. You can make it a practice to stretch frequently throughout the day. This releases toxins from your body, maintains flexibility, and slows down the aging process.

Regular exercise keeps muscles, including the heart muscle, in good working order. A good fast paced walk of 30 to 40 minutes, four times a week is all that is needed.

COUNSELING

Counseling may be of benefit to help uncover and release the roots of stress. Marital or family counseling may be helpful. Workshops and support groups that teach ways to handle stress, anger, communication difficulties, grief, loss, and other topics can be very beneficial but only if the counselor or group understands the importance of biochemical repair.

Counseling or therapy will be much more effective when your brain chemistry has had some time to begin rebalancing and you are used to your new nutritional routines. To clarify, I'm suggesting that you wait approximately six weeks after beginning this program in order to get the most out of counseling or therapy. Good support is always beneficial.

MERIDIAN TAPPING

Also known as Emotional Freedom Techniques, (EFT), this is the fastest growing Energy Psychology in the world. It is so powerful that it is now being *successfully* used with veterans suffering from PTSD (Post Traumatic Stress Disorder).

Dr. Joseph Mercola *states "Without a doubt meridian tapping techniques are the single most consistent and effective intervention in improving one's health that I have ever witnessed in over three decades of studying health."*[1]

Meridian Tapping consists of tapping on specific acupuncture sites around the head and upper chest while repeating phrases or while simply talking about emotional subjects. Very quickly, the emotional "charge" surrounding the issue is released. Layers upon layers of inner blockages are comfortably released in a very short time. You can learn about this technique by going to the web site www.EFTuniverse.com.

RESPONSIBILITY

While dysfunctional brain chemistry may be the root cause of negative behaviors and poor health, it doesn't release us from being responsible for the effects of our behavior on others.

FORGIVENESS and AMENDS

We owe it to our loved ones and friends to own any suffering we may have intentionally or unintentionally caused them and ask for their forgiveness. Whether they forgive us, or not, doesn't matter. What does matter is that we own our negative actions and forgive ourselves.

Attempt to make such amends as are appropriate and are welcomed by the other person(s). As always, do no harm to yourself or to others. When you have sincerely asked for forgiveness and offered amends, you've done your part. If they want to continue to harbor negativity, that's their choice. Don't continue to engage in their drama.

Once you have made these efforts, let the past go and move on. Move forward with hope, expectation of goodness in your life, and a sparkle in your eye.

SUPPORT

Asking for and accepting support while on the road to improving your health is of utmost importance. I can't stress that enough. In addition to emotional support, there are many alternative therapies that can be extremely beneficial.

SOME SUGGESTED ALTERNATIVE THERAPIES

(There are too many to list them all.)

REIKI	ACUPUNCTURE
YOGA	NATUROPATHIC
TAI CHI	MUSIC THERAPY
QIGONG	AROMA THERAPY
MASSAGE	ENERGY HEALING
FENG SHUI	QUANTUM TOUCH®
DRUMMING	MERIDIAN TAPPING
BIOFEEDBACK	NEURO-LINGUISTICS
HOMEOPATHY	THERAPEUTIC TOUCH
REFLEXOLOGY	AURICULAR THERAPY
CRANIAL-SACRAL THERAPY	CHIROPRACTIC ADJUSTMENT
BRAIN STATE CONDITIONING	MYOFASCIAL TRIGGER POINT

Be patient. Respect your brain and body. They know what to do when given the proper ingredients to work with. Take some deep breaths, smile, and know you are on your way to a healthier life.

1 *Discover the Power of Meridian Tapping,* Patricia Carrington, PhD, 2008, Book Jacket

BEHAVIORAL DISORDERS & AD(H)D

Delinquency, crime and violence have steadily increased throughout our nation's history. We spend billions of dollars a year on law enforcement. We have the world's largest prison population. Approximately 1 in every 31 American adults is in prison, on parole, or on probation.

Dr. William Walsh, PhD, is an internationally recognized expert in the field of nutritional medicine. Over 30 years he developed biochemical treatments for patients with behavioral disorders, ADHD, autism, depression, anxiety disorders, schizophrenia, and Alzheimer's disease that are used by doctors throughout the world.

The following information is taken from his recently released book *Nutrient Power – Heal Your Biochemistry And Heal Your Brain.*

For over 100 years we have operated on the belief that violent criminals are created by flawed life circumstances – poverty, child abuse, bad parenting, and broken homes. Of course these circumstances influence one's behavior but the underlying cause is usually bad brain chemistry.

Behavioral disorders usually show up before the age of four. When these children are identified and treated biochemically, the results are healthy and normal teens and adults. Once they are past the age of 14, Dr. Walsh found it was usually too difficult to repair brain chemistry because people were too addicted to substances or too oppositional to accept treatment.

AD(H)D – ATTENTION DEFICIT HYPERACTIVITY DISORDER

About 50% of the children treated by Dr. Walsh for behavioral disorders were also diagnosed with a learning disability or with ADHD. Biochemical treatment with these children had good results.

AD(H)D is an umbrella term given to several different learning disorders. Dr. Walsh's chemical data base of 5,600 cases indicated that 75% of these persons also had a history of a significant behavioral disorder. Left untreated, the genetic, or genetically influenced, tendencies will persist throughout life. While environmental factors have an influence upon the disorder, clearly brain chemistry is equally important.

The result of years of research with thousands of cases has proven that correcting brain chemistry with micronutrients and nutrition can positively change the lives of these children, and of course, of their families. If the condition is inherited, then the family will also benefit from brain chemistry repair. I recommend Dr. Walsh's book to those who are looking for in-depth research and results.

AD(H)D & ALCOHOL ADDICTION

According to David Miller, author of *Overload – Attention Deficit Disorder and the Addictive Brain*, it is probable that from 50% to 70% of alcoholics have undiagnosed AD(H)D. The Post Acute Withdrawal Syndrome (PAWS) that affects almost all recovering alcoholics is identical to AD(H)D symptoms. A high level of both internal and external stress leads to quick relapse. These symptoms are reduced or eliminated with a biochemical approach to alcohol recovery, which greatly increases recovery rates.

For more information read *How to Quit Drinking For Good and Feel Good – The NEW Alcoholism Story* by Suka Chapel-Horst RN, PhD. This book is available on the web site www.AriseAlcoholRecovery.com, www.Amazon.com, and through national booksellers.

BEHAVIORS

Barbara Reed Stitt, PhD, in her work with hundreds of probationers with criminal histories, discovered six consistent patterns. [See Note]

1. No breakfast.
2. High consumption of sugar and other refined carbohydrates.
3. High consumption of processed foods.
4. Low consumption of lean proteins.
5. Low consumption of fresh fruits and vegetables.
6. High milk consumption.

Studies showed that children who got into trouble with the law drank almost twice as much milk as children who were not lawbreakers. Allergies to milk are related to many of the challenging behaviors of children, beginning in infancy if the child is not breast fed, or from breast milk if the mother is using drugs or has allergies.

Today we see mothers giving young children boxes of juice thinking that it's a healthy choice. In fact, it's really feeding sugar to the young child, creating a potent addiction and hypoglycemia. Giving candy, sweets, and sodas to children isn't a treat. It's drugging them. Fast food meals are creating fatal results. Because we don't see the physical effects immediately, or don't recognize the source of the behavioral effects, we think we are doing them a favor.

Perhaps the shenanigans of our adult politicians were fed to them in their childhood. We are creating the world of the future by how we feed and educate our children while they are small.

NOTE: Read *Food and Behavior* by Barbara Reed Stitt, PhD. This book can be ordered from www. BrainworksRecovery.com.

PART THREE

Let Your Spirit Soar
Resources For Daily Living

PARACHUTES - RESOURCES FOR DAILY LIVING

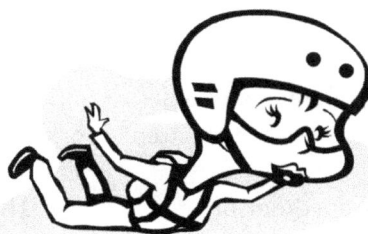

We have, within us, all the psychological resources we need to accomplish our desires. I call these resources, "parachutes". Like parachutes, these resources guide us safely toward physical, emotional, and mental grounding, while allowing us to experience the joy of soaring freely.

In the past, we may not have always tapped into those resources and sometimes they may have seemed to elude us, but they are there. In this part of the book, you'll learn some methods for tapping into your inner resources, allowing you to respond more usefully to life situations, with the result that your desires and goals will more naturally and easily materialize in your life.

Positive thinking begets positive results. Negative thinking begets negative results. We've all known people who seem to think and talk negatively most of the time. They believe, or fear, that things aren't going to work out right and they expect the worst. Their life seems to bear out their expectations. They have a constant stream of "bad luck", which only serves to reinforce their ongoing negativity. In fact, they have actually drawn the "bad luck" to themselves by focusing and concentrating their emotional and mental energy on their fears.

Positive thinking people, on the other hand, have entirely different outcomes. They attract to themselves all manner of good fortune. It doesn't matter if a person is "good" or "bad". It's not about whether people deserve something good in their lives. It's about their expectations and what they are focusing their mental and feeling-energy upon.

So what do we do when we experience negative emotions, emotions that make us mad, sad, or scared? All emotions are normal. They occur, automatically, in response to the sights, sounds, smells, tastes, and what we physically feel, combined with our history and individual belief system. However, we don't have to wallow in the negative emotions.

Sadness and depression, as the result of loss, death, and unwanted happenings, is normal. However, when the depression turns into a chronic condition, unrelieved over time, either a biochemical imbalance or unconscious beliefs are the culprit. (See Chapter 44.)

Once we recognize and feel negative emotions, they have served their purpose which is to alert us to the fact that something needs attention. We are most *resourceful* when we are not perceiving life through the filter of emotions. When we step outside our emotions, we have the opportunity to recognize useful information giving us the opportunity to tap into our inner resources and come up with the most appropriate and comfortable responses to deal with life situations.

The exercises you are going to read about can be quickly effective because they work with the unconscious, not conscious mind. They work with the Reward Pathway, the same part of the brain that is responsible for addictions, moods, depression, and all the symptoms we've been addressing in the first two parts of this book.

Instead of thinking about life as being filled with "obstacles", think about the "opportunities" we are given to learn and grow. I hope you will take the time to explore and benefit from these seventeen "parachutes". Your health will soar to new heights when you do, I promise. I know because I have been flying ever since I learned about these practices.

If some of these resources seem unusual at first, it's only because they are new and different from what you may have known before. However, if we want different outcomes in our life, we have to do something different to get them. Do you want to continue the same practices that aren't working very well for you? What does that do for you?

Take a leap of faith, as I did when I jumped out of an airplane at 18,000 feet and experienced a glorious sense of freedom and joy and just plain fun. You don't have to go that far. In fact, just using these exercises can make a huge difference in your ability to respond more effectively to life's events.

These resources may be done alone or with another person. If you have someone else read the directions to you, you will be able to just focus on what you are doing. Find a partner to share these resources with. You will come to love them as you experience their many very real benefits. You don't have to do them all. Pick out the ones that work for you.

I wish for you, good health, happiness, and many blessings as you explore and enjoy these life-expanding parachutes.

REPTILIAN COMPLEX AND STRESS REDUCTION

As a prelude to "soaring" let me introduce you to the most primitive part of the brain, the reptilian complex, the same brain that's in reptiles. It lies, highly protected, deep within the brain stem and its sole purpose is to keep us alive by maintaining the status quo.

Our "reptilian brain" keeps all physical functions operating within the range necessary for survival, including heartbeat, breathing, sleep, and hunger patterns.

We emotionally experience this as a need for some degree of ritual and repetition. While these needs differ from person to person, they are a necessary requirement for survival. (This is one of the reasons why autistic children rock their bodies.) We have daily routines and habit patterns. We drive the same routes to our destinations, frequent favorite restaurants and are comforted by religious or spiritual rituals, for example. These repetitious behaviors, no matter what they are, satisfy our primitive, reptilian brain, making it feel safe, and, as a result, reduce our physical stress levels.

Some people are more uncomfortable with change than others. When too much change puts stress on the "reptile", our physical, emotional, and mental health will be compromised.

When you feel overwhelmed or stressed out, besides taking the aminos, do some repetitive actions to sooth the reptilian brain. Mowing, ironing, rocking, rowing, exercising, walking, dancing, drumming, or swinging, for example. Let it be mindless and repetitious movement. If you keep your reptile happy, you will be happier, too. How simple is that?

ALL ABOUT BREATHING

PARACHUTE #1

Releases self-limiting emotions.
Accesses feelings of calmness and peace.
Increases resourcefulness and mental clarity.
Helps to tell the difference between emotions and hunger/full signals.

DEEP BREATHING

Most people usually breathe high in their chest cavity with short, irregular breaths. This kind of breathing stimulates nerve endings that cause the brain to send hormones throughout the body resulting in worry, anxiety, and fear. However, when we breathe deeply into our lungs, allowing the diaphragm to move down and our rib cage and abdomen to expand, we stimulate another set of nerve endings which permit the brain to emit a different set of chemicals, causing us to become relaxed, calm, and peaceful or more mentally alert. With practice we can change our emotional state in seconds.

FINDING YOUR CENTER OF GRAVITY

Place your thumb on your navel. Then place your index finger two inches below it on your abdomen. Your physical center of gravity lies in the center of your body, behind your index finger. Imagine that there is a balloon in this area, or a ball, of a golden-orange color. Visualize it glowing brightly. (Orange is the color of vibrant, glowing, good health.)

ABDOMINAL BREATHING – For relaxation and calmness

Place one hand on your abdomen and the other hand on the side of your rib cage, to feel these movements more easily. BREATH IN while allowing your abdomen and lower rib cage to EXPAND. Then BREATH OUT allowing your abdomen and rib cage to MOVE IN.

If you are having trouble with this, lie flat on your back. You'll notice that you are breathing perfectly, naturally, just as babies do!

As you breathe in, visualize the air being drawn down into the golden-orange ball in your abdomen. You may pretend you are blowing up a balloon there. Of course we know our lungs aren't in our abdomen but the act of visualizing in this manner helps us to completely fill the lungs. As you release the breath, imagine it to be flowing out all the way from your center of gravity in the abdomen to your mouth. Continue to bring the air down into your center of gravity and begin to count as you breathe.

Rhythm

1. First, release all the air from your lungs. Then breathe in SLOWLY AND EVENLY to a mental count of four. Count: "In… Two… Three… Four…" as you draw the breath DEEPLY down into the golden-orange ball in your abdomen. Take in just as much air at each count of four as you did on the count of one.
2. Now, SLOWLY AND EVENLY, *release* the breath for another count of four. Count: "Out… Two… Three… Four…". Just as much breath should be leaving your body at the count of four as was leaving at the count of one.
3. Repeat Steps 1 and 2.

Chest Breathing

Breathing high in the chest stimulates anxiety. Do not allow your shoulders to rise. (If they do, you're not breathing deeply into your abdomen.) You can watch yourself in a mirror by facing frontwards. Then turn and watch yourself breathe as you face to the side. Men tend to be natural abdominal breathers.

Hyperventilation

At first, if you are not in the habit of deep breathing, you may hyperventilate. Simply adjust the amount of air you breathe in to feel comfortable while maintaining a steady flow of air for the full four counts.

Pace

Begin breathing at a comfortable pace. Then slow the pace to one count per second. At 60 counts per minute, your heartbeat will soon slow down to that most healthy pace and you will become relaxed, peaceful and calm. Continue until you feel wonderful.

Hunger or Craving Signals Versus Emotional Responses

With abdominal breathing, excessive emotions will be calmed. If you're still getting hunger or craving signals after breathing a few minutes, it will be true hunger or craving signals, not emotional reactions. It's time for healthy food or your brain-satisfying aminos, whichever is most appropriate.

Extra Benefit – Induce Sleep

This is an excellent method to quickly induce sleep at bedtime.

Adding Pictures

It's important to keep your mind focused on the experience of breathing and the count. To keep other thoughts from entering into your thinking, you can add relaxing, enjoyable imagery.

You might imagine ocean waves building up to a peak, rolling onto the shore, then receding back into the ocean. You can OBSERVE the waves, or you can BECOME the waves as you feel yourself slowly filling and then releasing the breath.

You might visualize an open window with a breeze blowing the curtains into the room and then drawing them out of the window.

Or you might observe a swing, or feel yourself to be on a swing, moving forward and backward with your inhalations and exhalations.

Any imagery that works for you will give your breathing an added dimension for releasing negative emotions, increasing calmness and mental clarity.

DIAPHRAGMATIC BREATHING – For Mental Clarity

Follow Steps 1 and 2, as with the abdominal breathing. However, this time, hold your **abdominal wall firm** so that it doesn't expand with the inhalation. Instead, allow the diaphragm to **expand the lower rib cage** outward, even further.

Instead of focusing on the golden-orange ball in your abdomen, focus on the lower rib cage, letting it fill completely with oxygen. This will improve your alertness and mental clarity.

SUMMARY

FOR RELAXATION AND CALMNESS

BREATHE IN;
Lower rib cage AND abdomen
EXPAND

BREATHE OUT:
Lower rib cage AND abdomen become
SMALLER

FOR MENTAL CLARITY

HOLD ABDOMEN FIRM

BREATHE IN;
Lower rib cage EXPANDS

BREATHE OUT:
Lower rib cage becomes SMALLER

PRACTICE PERFECTS

If you practice regularly, several times every day, for about two months, your body will automatically begin to breathe this way most of the time. You might notice how much calmer you are becoming more of the time. It will be due to the changes in your brain chemistry as a result of regular deep breathing.

Do the breathing at least twice a day for ten minutes each session. Sit up for your practice sessions versus lying down. (It's very easy to fall asleep when lying down.) Also do the breathing exercise while you drive, shower, or perform any mundane tasks which don't require conscious attention elsewhere. Remember to think only about the count. If your mind wanders to other thoughts you will lose focus. Keep it simple and boring and if you are a visual person, add the imagery.

Breathe deeply whenever you notice yourself becoming too emotional or when you want to discover if you are really experiencing hunger or craving signals versus excess emotional energy.

Abdominal breathing will become automatic in about two months if you concentrate on training your brain every day. The result will be a life of VITALITY, CLEARER THINKING, INCREASED HEALTH and GREATLY REDUCED STRESS REACTIONS. It is truly *breathing for life*.

THE HIDDEN PERSUADER
COLOR BREATHING

PARACHUTE #2

Releases tension and stress.
Decreases anger and irritability.
Creates peace and harmony within.

Science has long known that color is a powerful and important resource for health – physical, emotional and mental. I'm not talking about the colors people choose to wear based upon their skin and hair coloring. The Quick Color Code shows the UNCONSCIOUS PSYCHOLOGICAL effects that color has upon us.

You can test this by imagining that you are in a room with no windows. Visualize the floor, walls, and ceiling completely painted with a color. Imagine that you are standing in the center of that room. See and feel the color surrounding you. Notice the physical response of your body, as well as your emotional response, and your mental state.

Of course every color has many shades and hues. You can have even more fun by remaining in your imaginary room while slightly and gradually changing the shade and brightness of that same color. You will notice a changing response to the color changes.

Having this knowledge permits you to have a powerful ally in managing your emotions, stress levels, and mental clarity, even affecting your ability to go to sleep.

The Quick Color Code that follows gives you an idea of what specific colors do. There are over nine million shades of color, so when you think of a color, remember that each one has a broad spectrum. Shades, hues, brightness, and luminosity all affect that color. Trust your instinct. As you think of the color you might want for its relaxing or healing properties, notice how it feels. Not right? Change the color until you find just the right one.

QUICK COLOR CODE

BLACK: Chaos, mystery, power.
WHITE: Truth, purity, honesty, best healing color. (Contains all colors.)
SILVER: Mental sharpness, unemotional.
GOLD: Emotional warmth, profound.
RED: Intensifies, stimulator, energizer big time! Fast energy.
ORANGE: For general good health, energizer, lifts spirits, comfortable. Stimulates appetite!
BROWN: Mentally relaxing, grounded.
PINK: Caring, kindness, romantic love.
MAUVE: Compassion, spiritual love.
GREEN: Relaxes eyes, flexible, ongoing energy for mental concentration, and focus. Soothing energy. Healing color.
GREEN: Camouflage green – Death.
YELLOW: Stimulates concrete, detail-thinking, cheerful, non-invasive energy.
BLUE: Light blue is creative, expressive, safety.
INDIGO: Physiologically resting and releasing. Emotional cleansing.
PURPLE: Spiritual and mystical or sexual and hallucinatory.
VIOLET: Tolerant, accepting, seeking. Highest spiritual color.

COLOR BREATHING

Think of a color that carries the feeling you want in your body. Imagine breathing in air of that color and imagine it circulating throughout your body, filling every molecule and space within the sub-atomic particles of your body.

If you have areas of tension, send the color to those specific areas. Imagine the tension evaporating out through your skin as a gray or black cloud. Fill the space where the tension was with the color of your choice. Continue to breathe the color until the muscles relax and you are feeling calmer.

Within five minutes of exposure to any color, there will usually be physical, emotional, and mental changes. This is not a psychological reaction. It's the body's natural response to the *electro-magnetic qualities* of color in the light spectrum. The body responds just as easily to imagined color as to external visualized color.

GROUP BREATHING

Next time you are involved in a heated discussion, suggest everyone interrupt the talk briefly for some deep breathing.

Cooperation and conflict-resolution can follow more easily when the emotions are calmed and mental clarity is restored.

30

TORNADO

PARACHUTE #3

*Clears and releases negativity received
from both yourself and from others.*

VISUALIZATION

Some of the following resources use imaginative visualizations. This process is extremely important because imagery is the most important language of the brain.

In the other-than-conscious mind, which is where all change takes place, images, sounds, and feelings are how the brain thinks. Words and numbers don't compute in this area of the brain except as symbols which then call up the images, sounds, and feelings.

By the way, if you think you don't visualize, just PRETEND how you think the image would look. That's good enough.

Actually, everyone visualizes. Some people, however, are so good at it, and so quick, that the image is gone before it's really noticed. All you have to do, if you are one of those super-quick visualizers, is to slow down the image so you can see it more easily or just imagine and *feel* it there.

BOUNDARIES

For years psychologists have talked about the need for healthy "boundaries". That means being able to say "no" and not allowing others to control your behavior and emotions. It means not becoming enmeshed in other people's "stuff". It means moving toward self-dependency versus too much co-dependency. It doesn't mean lack of love. It means respect for both yourself and others. It means taking self responsibility for your responses and actions and giving others the same right for themselves.

How do you know what the right boundaries are? You can spend years trying to figure that one out. Yet, in just seconds, you can use the following resources of the Tornado, Shield, Bubble and Color Protection and your boundary is automatically there. Your other-than-conscious mind already knows exactly where your most healthy boundary ought to be. It simply places the boundary where it will be the most useful for you.

If there doesn't seem to be a valid reason for your sudden moodiness or negativity, assess the people around you to see whether you are feeling what THEY are feeling. If so, you need to 1) RELEASE their emotions (and your own negative reactions) and 2) PROTECT yourself from the invasion of further negative emotions from others.

TORNADO

1. Visualize, about SIX inches above your head, the funnel of a white tornado cloud. The widest, upper part of the funnel is about nine inches wider than the circumference of your body. The lower, narrow end is the diameter of a quarter.
2. Now, with your eyes closed (to decrease distractions), visualize pulling the small end of the funnel down through the top of your head and into your body.
3. Imagine this funnel is whirling in a clockwise motion. This means it is rotating from your right shoulder to your back, to your left shoulder and around to the front of your body. As the narrow end of the funnel moves downward through your body, the wider portion swirls outside your body. You may even sense the movement around you.
4. Continue to pull this funnel cloud down, through and around your body. It is drawing the negative energies into it. At times it may seem to slow down, or not want to move as fast as you are imagining it. Wait for the image to follow your thinking. The tornado will not automatically flow through your body. If you stop the concentration, it will cease.
5. Pull the funnel-cloud down between your legs and send it thirty feet into the earth. Visualize the negative energies being cleansed by the earth and returning to the universe in their pure and natural state.
6. Repeat as necessary

This tornado-funnel may be used as frequently as necessary to cleanse both your inner and outer space. You can even do it while in the presence of others. They won't notice.

COLOR PROTECTION

PARACHUTE #4

*Protects from emotions
and negativity of others.*

To protect yourself from future invasion of negative thoughts and emotions, you'll place a mental shield around yourself. This won't stop the negative thoughts YOU create but it will shield you from the negativity of OTHERS. First, use the Tornado exercise to cleanse your space. Then you're ready to protect it.

1. Close your eyes and visualize or feel the presence of a star, or sun, about TWELVE inches above your head. Imagine this star or sun sending out a luminous, PURPLE-VIOLET light, like the blue color in a gas flame, with some purple added. Draw this light down into the top of your head and down through your body.

2. Continue to draw this light into yourself, letting it circulate through all the muscles, tissues, and organs. Visualize and feel it moving into the cellular structures and through the wall of each molecule. See it moving into the spaces within the atoms themselves.

3. Now imagine the purple-violet light expanding out through your pores and into the space around yourself. In addition to filling your body, let it flow around you, creating an outer-egg of purple-violet luminous light. The electro-magnetic energy of the purple/violet light protects your boundaries. It forms a shell, if you will, that will deflect negative energies from entering your personal space.

4. Again, return your imagination to that star or sun you created earlier above your head. This time, imagine a beautiful luminous GOLDEN-YELLOW light coming down into the top of your head. As before, draw this light through your body, into each muscle, the blood vessels, the organs and all the tissues of the body. Visualize it moving through the walls of each cell and into the atoms of your body. See and feel yourself filled with the light. Now imagine this golden-yellow light moving out through the pores of your skin. It pushes the purple-violet light further out as the golden-yellow fills both your body and the space about you

inside the purple-violet surrounding you. The electro-magnetic energy of the Golden/Yellow light brings mental clarity to your mind.

5. Return again to the star or sun, twelve inches above your head, and this time draw into your head a BRIGHT PEARLIZED WHITE light. Draw this light down into your body as you did with the previous colors. And again, let it fill up your entire body right down into the space within each atom. Feel the pulsating energy of the light. The electro-magnetic-energy of the Pearlized White light creates a higher vibration that puts you in touch with your Higher Self, your Soul, a Higher Power, Spirit, Source, Presence, or any name of God you resonate to. It encourages freedom from limitations and openness to new awarenesses.

6. Now, as you allow this pearlized white light to remain within your body, let it also expand outward through the pores of your skin. You are now filled with pearlized white light which also extends outside your body. The white light is surrounded, on its outside, by golden-yellow light. That golden-yellow light, in turn, is surrounded with purple-violet light.

If you have difficulty visualizing the colors, just pretend you are putting the colors in place and feel their energy. Your brain will still get the message.

From the outside it looks like a purple-violet egg, lined with gold and filled with pearlized white that both surrounds and fills your body. The egg fills about nine inches to three feet of space around you, including the ground under your feet. You can even surround your car to protect it when you are driving. I put it around airplanes when I'm flying and around my motor home, and house.

TIMING

Do this every morning and evening for three days to build a strong image. The effects are cumulative, like building a snow-ball. After three days, do this every morning and the energies will stay with you until the next day. In fact, if you miss a day, the effects will remain for awhile if you've been building the image strongly each day. If you quit, however, the protection will wear off and you'll have to start over with extra time, morning and night, to re-establish its strength.

FREQUENCY

This can be used at any time you feel an urge to protect yourself. It can't be overdone nor can it ever hurt you or any other person. If you stop using this for awhile, you may notice increasing stress and will later re-establish the protection because the benefits will have become obvious.

MENTAL CHALLENGES

If you are in a situation which calls for meeting intense MENTAL conflict, visualize GOLDEN specks, or sparkles, within the WHITE LIGHT. The sparkles are like those thrown off by Fourth of July sparklers, or the dancing sparkles seen on a shimmering lake. This image will keep you more mentally balanced.

EMOTIONAL CHALLENGES

If you are in a situation which calls for meeting intense EMOTIONAL conflict, visualize SILVER specks, or sparkles, within the WHITE light. This image will help to keep you calm.

BOTH EMOTIONAL AND MENTAL CHALLENGES

Just fill your space with both GOLDEN and SILVER sparkles together.

32

SHIELD

PARACHUTE #5

Protects you from negative emotions and
confrontation that is directed specifically at you.

1. Create an image of a Plexiglas shield in front of you. Make it taller and wider than your body. Place it on the ground and allow it to rise above your head. Imagine it to be three to four inches thick and made of bullet-proof material. Place this shield directly in front of you about two feet away from you. If you have difficulty visualizing the shield, just *pretend* you have put it there. Knowing you have done that, continue with the process.

2. You can see and hear perfectly through the shield. Feelings of sincere love, caring, and kindness flow easily through it. But it has the wonderful quality of shielding out all the *negative* emotions of others. When others are putting out negative energy, the energy strikes the shield and returns back to the sender, where it belongs. You are protected. Likewise, you are equally protected when someone is confronting you directly. This may sound like a Walt Disney scenario, but I assure you, it works. This imagery is the language of the brain and of the other-than-conscious mind, along with sounds and feelings.

3. There is a little one-way door in the shield with a lock on the inside which only you control. Only you know where this door is.

4. Now, just in case you've already picked up someone else's negative emotions, imagine opening the one-way door. COMMAND your unconscious mind to send all the feelings that don't belong to you out through the door and right back to their source.

5. You can also focus upon a specific emotion, thought, or physical feeling you wish to release, then make the following statement. "If this be mine I accept responsibility for it. If it is not mine, *BE GONE FROM ME NOW!!*" Speak or think this statement with firmness and decisiveness.

6. You might FEEL the negativity moving out of you through the one-way door, you might HEAR it moving away, or you might even SEE the negativity going back to its source. You might see a cloud, or strings,

or little particles going out the door. One person saw little penguins marching right out the door. Or you might hear a "whoosing" sound, or the sound of little feet pattering away, or the sound of a dump truck emptying itself out. You may want to *blow* the emotions out the door.

7. You'll feel more spacious inside, or lighter when the unwanted emotion(s) are released. Your experience is uniquely your own and may be different from these. That's just fine.

8. When you hear, see, or feel all the negative emotions you took on from another person have been released, close and lock your one-way door. What you are left with will be your own feelings. Allow them to fill up the empty space and know that this is you.

No one else can see or feel your shield. It's your secret. Just zap it up in front of you whenever you need it. You can imagine the shield, instantly, in any setting. Put it up when you're confronted by anger, frustration, irritability, or any emotions others are experiencing that you don't want. The feelings of others belong to them. They need all their feelings in order to know themselves and take responsibility for who they are and how they experience life.

Be honest and don't steal the feelings of others.

33

BUBBLE

PARACHUTE #6

*Protects you from unknown negativity that might be
bombarding you from anywhere in your environment.*

This exercise fulfills the same function as the shield but in this case it fully surrounds you like being inside the shell of an egg. The shield curves under your feet and over your head. Made of the same bullet-proof Plexiglas material, with its own secret one-way door, it shields you from negative emotions coming from anywhere around and about you that you might not even be aware of. The BUBBLE can be useful in a large gathering of people (a conference, shopping mall, or state fair) or in a room where the atmosphere doesn't feel "right" to you such as when a "gripe" session is going on around you.

To Build the Bubble (One Time Only):

1. Stand up, hold out your hands and feel the inside of your bubble from top to bottom and all around the inside. It's like being a mime and describing the image with your hands. Actually, physically doing this helps your mind to implant the image into the kinesthetic memory of your body, making it an even more powerful and useful tool.
2. Feel the texture (smooth or rough) and temperature (warm or cool).
3. Turn around inside the bubble and feel, with your hands, its entire shape from above your head to around your feet.

To Use the Bubble:

Just quickly imagine the bubble around you and it is there. (You don't have to "feel" it with your hands again. It's already in your kinesthetic memory.)

Have fun using these imaginary visualizations. The other-than-conscious mind doesn't understand the words, "I don't want to take on the feelings of other people." It *does* understand the protective *image*, which gives the same message in a way the brain *can* understand. In Japan you have to speak Japanese to get your message across. Now you're learning how to speak Brain Language. Good for you.

NEUTRAL OBSERVER SHIELD

PARACHUTE #7

*Permits you to experience your own
emotions without being controlled by them.
Increases objectivity and resourcefulness.*

Put up your Plexiglas shield and imagine seeing yourself on the other side of it. You are objectively seeing you, as you are, over there. If you can't *see* yourself, just *pretend* there is an image of yourself on the other side of the shield. Now, open the one-way door and send all YOUR feelings through the door over to the you that is on the other side of the shield. Notice, particularly, the way I use words in the example below.

Example:

I project an image of myself over to the other side of the shield. Then I *tell* my unconscious mind to send all of *my* feelings over to Suka. I see, hear and/or feel those feelings moving over to Suka even though I don't know just WHAT those feelings might be, specifically. I observe Suka, objectively and unemotionally. I observe her, over there, with HER emotions, while I, over here, get in touch with all my knowledge, experience, and intuition to help me resourcefully come up with ideas which might be useful to Suka, over there.

NOTE: Suka is on the other side of the shield and "I" am here.

This "I" is my neutral, objective self, free of emotions, who can see and hear, but not *feel* because Suka over there has all the emotions. In this manner, I recognize, accept and honor, NOT DENY, how Suka is feeling, without being encumbered by the limitations of excessive emotions. Thus, I can be more resourceful and objective, able to come up with useful solutions to whatever is causing the emotions.

HUNGER CHECK SHIELD

PARACHUTE #8

*To discover if body signals are caused by
emotions, appetite triggers or real hunger.*

How can we know whether our body is truly hungry or whether we're just over-stressed and emotional? Here's a way to use your SHIELD to find out.

1. Put up your two to four inch thick Plexiglas SHIELD, floor to ceiling and wall to wall. Send an image of yourself over to the other side of it.
2. Tell your unconscious mind to send all your feelings through the one-way door to the image of you on the other side. Wait until all of the feelings are gone from you and are over there.
3. Now notice whether you feel emotionally neutral, the observer you experienced in Resource #7. Emotions will transfer to the image, however, hunger pangs won't transfer. So, if you still experience the urge to eat, your body is probably truly in need of nourishment. Go for it.

COLOR STATE CHANGE

PARACHUTE #9

Creates a state of resourcefulness.
Stimulates an attitude change.
Reduces the stress in stressful situations.

1. Think of the present stressful situation. What would you like to feel instead of what you are currently feeling? What inner resources would be useful to help you cope with the stress? Inner resources are confidence, calmness, curiosity, humor, focus, concentration, energy, organization, motivation, persistence, mental quickness, dexterity, empowerment, trust, understanding, caring, etc.

2. Now think of a situation where you had the resource(s) you desire. Remember a situation from the past or make one up where that resource is present.

3. When you have that situation in mind, mentally step into it and experience it fully. While you are experiencing the desired resource, ask yourself, "If there were a color that would give me this same feeling, what would it be?" When you know the color that would give you the same feeling, let the image go.

4. Now, test the color. Just pretend there is a small neon tube running down the center of your body. Into the top of that tube, pour your color. If you have more than one color, let them swirl around each other or flow side by side. (If you mix the colors they become muddy.) Then let the color(s) radiate throughout your entire body, filling up all the molecules, going all the way into the atomic spaces of your body, or imagine the color as if it were a cloud that fills and surround you.

5. Check whether this color gives you the feeling of the resource you desired. If it doesn't, let the light go out. Flush out the neon tube with clear light as if it were water. Return to the situation that carried the resource(s) you wanted and check to see what other color will give you the feeling you desire. Repeat the neon tube check.

6. When the color gives you the feeling of the resource you desire, then KEEPING THAT FEELING, think of the situation that was originally giving you stress. Bring that DESIRED resource-color with you to the stressful situation and notice how your perception of the situation changes, reducing the stress level so you can cope with it more usefully. Keep feeling yourself filled with the color and you'll keep the desired resource.

Example: You're experiencing a time crunch. Piles of paper on the desk in front of you need your immediate attention. Someone comes to you and insists you have to take on another project, right now! You think, "It's too much. I don't have time. I can't do it. But I must. Blah. Blah. Blah." The stress is making your body tense, your head aches, there's a lump in your throat, your stomach feels upset, on and on. You know!

Close your eyes or look somewhere else. Think about what you'd like to be feeling right now. What feeling would let you be resourceful so that you could decide how to handle the situation. For this example, let's say you'd like a feeling of peace and calmness with just the right amount of energy to calmly do what has to be done. Great.

Now you let the image of your desk go away as you look into your memory. You might think of a time when you are walking along the ocean beach. You have a purposeful stride which makes your body feel energetic, yet flowing with the movement. You are enjoying the sun's warmth on your body and the sound of the surf. The rhythm of the waves is relaxing. You just let yourself become immersed in the image. Feel it completely. You are calm and peaceful, relaxed, yet energetic. (Or you make up an experience that has the resources you desire.)

When that feeling is flowing completely throughout your body, think of a color that gives you the same feeling. Take your time and let a color or colors come into your mind. Then let the image go.

Now test the color by pouring it into the imaginary neon tube down the center of your body. Let the color fill up your entire being and notice whether the color gives you the same feeling as the ocean image did. If not, go back to the image. Once again, get into the entire feeling. Then think of *another* color that would give you that feeling. Let the image go and repeat the color check by pouring the color into the tube and filling your body with it.

When you have the desired feeling in your body, maintain that state, bringing it to your desk. You notice, now, that you can decide how to handle your projects in a calm, relaxed, yet energetically flowing manner, just as you asked for.

NOTE: In the future, when you desire this same feeling, simply pour the color into your neon tube and let it fill your body while you fully integrate the feeling throughout your body and mental state. You don't have to access the original picture again, unless, of course, you want to.

If the color no longer "does it" for you, then go back to the original picture, or create another one, and choose the color(s) that will give the feeling of the resource you desire. Repeat the process.

The color state-change will work for any situation where you want to access more of your internal resources. This can be with relationships, your social and career life, or even changing to a more effective state for improving your sports abilities. Find the color that increases your motivation to perform those less desired tasks that "have" to be done. The strategy works whenever you want to change your internal state.

(Paint chips from a paint store can enhance your color visualizations.)

Now you can transform self-limiting emotions into resourcefulness.

MOVING PICTURES

PARACHUTE #10

(A) Releases unwanted thoughts from the mind.

If you'd like to be relieved of a thought that is an imagined worry about the future, create an image of the worry. Then make the image dimmer, duller, and smaller as you send it out into space. When the image is the size of a small dot, explode it into thousands of tiny pieces, letting them turn into ice crystals that melt and become completely absorbed in the universe. Now you can think about other things.

(B) Organizes thoughts.

Make individual images for each of the thoughts you want to organize in your mind. Perhaps you're trying to prioritize your tasks for the day. After you have an image of each one, create the image of a desktop.

Next, sort out the task images on your imaginary desktop. Then stack the images somewhere on the desktop where they will be out of your way, leaving only the image of the first task in front of you on that imaginary desktop.

The other tasks will still be there when you need them. You won't have to think about them until you are ready. When you are ready, just mentally put aside the finished task and bring the next task into place in front of you on the imaginary desktop. You'll find your mind is now orderly and will allow you to focus on the task at hand.

(C) Switches from unwanted to wanted thoughts.

Perhaps you're thinking of a sweet roll and can even see it in your mind. You would rather have an apple but the image of the sweet roll keeps popping up in front of you. Use the same process as in (A) to send the sweet roll into space, exploding and transforming it into the stuff of the universe.

Then, from somewhere in space see a tiny dot moving toward you getting bigger, brighter, and more colorful until you can make out that it's a shiny apple. Keep bringing the apple picture closer to you making it bigger, more colorful and brighter until you can't wait to get a real one and eat it. Then get one and eat it.

SUMMARY

Whenever you want to change from an "unwanted" thought to a "wanted" thought, first send the image of the unwanted thought out into space, watching it become dimmer, darker, and smaller until it becomes a small dot. Destroy the dot by any imaginary means that works for you. Then, from another distant small dark dot, bring forward the image of your "wanted" thought. Bring it right up in front of you, making it big and colorful.

You may have to repeat this a few times to release strong unwanted thoughts. After some practice, you'll be able to send away one thought while bringing the new on in, very swiftly, and even at the same time.

EDITING INTERNAL VIDEOS

PARACHUTE #11

Avoids self-sabotage.

How often do you find yourself visualizing negative consequences to future actions? I'll give you two very simple examples.

1. I hadn't worn high heels for some time. As I began to go down the stairs from the bedroom, I suddenly had a moving picture in my mind of myself tripping and falling all the way down those stairs.
2. I was alone on the stage, singing in front of a large audience when I suddenly forgot all of the words.

These pictures are a simple example of self-sabotage. Because our unconscious mind naturally seeks to *fulfill* our internal pictures, falling and forgetting my words, in the examples above, can occur very easily.

To decrease the likelihood of having the "worst" actually happen, you can simply...

EDIT YOUR INTERNAL VIDEOS! Here's how.

1. Stop what you are doing immediately when you have a negative thought and picture in your mind.
2. Notice clearly, exactly what you have just imaged in your mind.
3. Now, reverse the video or DVD, exactly as if you had your finger on a remote control that allows you to "run it backward". Remember how funny people look backing up, putting food back on their plate, lifting themselves back up onto the diving board?
4. When your internal video is reversed back to "start" (the beginning of your not-so-nice image) you can *edit* it. Now replay the scene as you WANT IT TO BE.
5. After the replay you can safely take action.

6. Examples:

   (a) I visualize myself "unfalling", very quickly, back *up* the stairs. Then I visualize myself walking safely down the stairs BEFORE I actually *do* walk down the stairs.

   (b) I visualize myself signing the song backwards, very quickly, all the way to the beginning. Then I visualize myself singing it perfectly to the end, and then I actually do sing it perfectly to the end.

That's all there is to it. Now, your unconscious won't sabotage you with the original negative action.

UNCONSCIOUS ALLY

PARACHUTE #12

*Increasing resourcefulness
when overwhelmed.*

When you are overwhelmed, call out the troops. Your vast and resourceful *unconscious self* is your ever-present ally. Even when you're ready to shut out the world and *mentally* escape, your hearing is still aware, your eyes are still registering information and your body is still responding to these senses. You can harness these sensory aspects of yourself and direct them to serve you well by taking over some of the tasks that are overwhelming you.

First, for the fun of it, just think about your unconsciousness as a part of you that handles all your memory, computes and sorts, as well as distorts and deletes all the information that comes into it. Think about that part of you as if it were a friend. (It is, if you treat it as such.) Ask that part of you what it wants to be called. Let it just throw up a name right out of the blue. My unconscious *demanded* to be called *Henry Henry the Third!* (No joke. He has a wonderful sense of humor.) Be sure to *thank* your unconscious for giving you its name and make friends with it.

Now the next time you feel overwhelmed, just TELL your unconscious ally to take in information, sort and categorize it, and to simply send you the information you need, when you need it. Then *you* go on with what you're doing. Having given the command to your unconscious, you can be assured it will follow your directions.

Example: Once when I was attending a workshop, I became so confused, lost, and frustrated that I noticed I was dozing instead of taking notes and listening carefully. I was overwhelmed. I simply told Henry Henry the Third to get all the information, understand it, sort it out, and give it to me whenever I needed to use it. Then I dozed off, on purpose.

A few weeks later, right when I needed to know that information and how to use it, I found everything I needed to know was right there in my conscious mind. It was as if I had never been confused. Henry Henry the Third had followed my instructions, to a "T," and listened while I dozed.

SECURITY BALANCE

PARACHUTE #13

*Puts ritual and regularity into your
life to meet your basic security needs.*

As much as 85% of our behavior can be motivated and directed by that Reptilian Complex you read about earlier. It's the instinctual brain whose entire and only mission is to meet our needs for survival. If we don't meet those needs, we will actually die, and if we aren't meeting those needs in healthy ways, we *will* meet them in *unhealthy* ways.

Because the instinctive brain is not conscious, and doesn't respond to our words (or thinking), we can help meet those needs constructively through repetitive actions that meet the instinctual brain's need for security. Any mundane activity that is PHYSICALLY ritualistic or has repetitive movements makes our instinctive brains happy. It's not intellectual stimulation that does it. It's the repetitive movements that count.

Shoveling snow, knitting, pounding nails, sawing wood, scrubbing the tub, ironing, crocheting, mowing the lawn, vacuuming, walking, swimming, rowing, square dancing, rocking in a rocking chair. Get the idea? Of course, if you have lots of *physical* repetition in your work, you may already have *too much* repetition, and need a little more *variety* in your life to break out of a rut.

Rituals such as yearly family reunions, weekly religious services, regular staff meetings, Saturday night movies or eating out, for example, also fill the need for security through repetition.

People have individual needs for ritual and repetition. Some need more than others. Regularly watching a weekly TV show, regular visits to a parent, set hairdresser appointment times, driving the same way to work every day, eating at the same restaurants, are fine ways to satisfy the reptile brain.

However, we can become so used to our rituals and so comfortable with them that we fail to expand and explore new and different ways of doing things. We may become overly comfortable and afraid of adventures that might take us out of our comfort zones.

It's healthy to take stock of our life choices in order to keep just the right balance between safety and security on the one hand, and exploration and expansion on the other.

For many years I dreamed of skydiving, of the feeling of soaring in the wind, of being free of the earth. I knew I would be exhilarated once I got out of the airplane. I also knew that I could never let go of the airplane door and make the jump. The thought terrified me.

I lived with these conflicting images for years. I even put a message on my answering machine that said I would return calls when I came back from skydiving. I knew I would never do it but I loved the idea of it. Most importantly, there was real feeling behind those images.

Much to my own amazement, one day I said I just might do it, after all. Before any door-clutching images took over, I reserved a date to take the leap with a nearby skydiving school. The date was set for about a week later. I focused on the wildness of it all, the craziness, the excitement, refusing to give in to images of fear. On the day I was to dive, the school informed me they didn't have enough students to take the plane up and they cancelled the dive. I could forget it and go home or come back the next day.

I was tempted to forget all about it, for sure. But I didn't want egg on my face, so I said I'd be back the next day and I was and I did skydive from 18,000 feet, the world's highest tandem skydive.

When it came time to jump out the airplane door, my heart was racing and I tried not to let fear overwhelm me. No need to worry. There is a saying that the skydiving instructor asks the student if he's ready to jump. If the student says "No", the instructor pushes him out the airplane door, later saying "I thought you said "Go". Well, it happened so fast. I wasn't allowed to stand in the door and think. Before I knew it, my co-jumper and I were dropping and somersaulting through the air and then stabilizing into a free fall at 120 miles an hour.

Long before the jump I had decided that if I ever did it, I would enjoy every moment. What's the point of wasting the time being scared? It wouldn't make any difference and would waste the precious experience. And I lived up to my decision, enjoying, exhilarating in the *expansion* of it.

For years I had feared the landing. The glider parachute made landing as gentle and easy as walking down a path. Of course, my jump partner was an experienced expert at all of it, making it one of the best experiences of my life. Yes, I will do it again.

I don't expect everyone to try skydiving, but I urge you to reach beyond your present edges. Expand your boundaries. Remove your limitations. When you do, as I did, you will gain more confidence in yourself, and have new perspectives on life. At the same time, maintain some of those healthy, ritualistic, survival behaviors for balance.

Play, have fun. Life is too serious to be taken seriously.

BELONGING BALANCE

PARACHUTE #14

Fills the need for belonging and being loved.

We can't depend upon others to meet our belonging needs, nor is it healthy to do so. Fortunately, there are healthy steps we can take to move from co-dependency to self-dependency.

To begin, nurture yourself. You are always there to meet your needs and you deserve to give yourself the time. Massage yourself, all over (when no one else is looking). The part of the brain that loves this doesn't know whose hands are doing the massage. It only knows it feels good and feels loved.

(Similarly, stroking comatose or unconscious persons can be helpful. Their mind may not "register" the soothing strokes, but their *body* knows and responds.)

If you don't' have a dog or cat, get a stuffed animal. Holding and petting it satisfies that same needy part of the brain that doesn't know the pet is stuffed. Kids know this. They rub teddy's ear on their nose and carry their blanket wherever they go. It works. When I was not married, I used to take a stuffed animal with me when I traveled. When I saw it propped up on the bed, always smiling at me, I laughed and felt great.

Lock the bathroom door and take a bubble bath, complete with candles, a soothing drink, a good junk book, and a big fluffy towel. Tell your family you're "out" for an hour. No phones and no interruptions and stick to it.

Just as some men like to get away on their hunting and fishing trips, or hole up in their man-caves with the guys, women need to get away with their female friends. Once or twice a year, go off for a weekend with your best women friends. Shop, walk, eat out, go to museums, the theater or movies, swim or golf, and best of all, stay up most of the night in your PJ's talking and giggling like high school girls. It's wonderful. No one understands a woman better than another woman. And, DON'T CALL HOME!

Go to a movie by yourself; eat out alone and people-watch or read. Go to the playground and swing. Read for pure escape. Even junk novels are great for losing yourself in fluff.

Give yourself gifts without guilt. Hunt for treasures, no matter how small, in antique stores, consignment shops, or Goodwill. Listen to uplifting audio cassettes, such as Wayne Dyer's *Excuses Begone!*. Purchase a magazine that you would normally forego.

Create wonderful, pleasant surroundings. (Most men have a harder time with this but they're trainable.) Have a fresh flower on your desk at work or table at home. Have toys (yes, toys) on your desk for break time; a top, rubber ball, train whistle. I have a Staples' *That's Easy* talking button, for example.

If people give you a hard time and you need to stand up for yourself more, take a course in assertiveness. You'll meet some nice people there. Don't let "caring friends" and "loving relatives" sabotage your optimal health goals.

Are you "friend" or "foe" towards yourself? You'll know you're on the right track when you enjoy being by yourself without being bored or feeling lonely. Mother Teresa said, "The greatest disease of [North Americans] is loneliness. But you always have you. Why not get to know and enjoy you?

JOURNEY TO THE CORE OF YOUR BEING

PARACHUTE #15

Letting go of the emotional and mental
"onion" layers that hide the real you.

There are many good self-help books available at your local book store. Support groups and individual counseling can be helpful. Take personal-growth workshops; go on retreats. Retreats can be for private time alone, outdoor activities, art classes, writing workshops, Outward Bound, or spiritual seeking. Some growth has to be done alone in the canyons of your mind. Some is done with another individual where listening and guidance are helpful. Some is done with a group of people in which there is the building of trust and acceptance. Each has its place.

The core of your being is a spiritual place where you get in touch with your own beautiful, higher self and goodness. It's the loving center of your being, and it leads to a wonderful special contact with resources greater than your conscious thinking self. Ask, seek, and knock; the door will surely be opened for you.

LOVE YOUR BODY NOW

PARACHUTE #16

*Gaining the cooperation of your
body for restoring optimal health.*

Be grateful for the innate ability your body has to change and respond to your needs in the most useful manner open to it at any given time.

If I insult you and then ask you to do something nice for me, I doubt if you will be inclined to help me. Why should you? Your body is similar. Hate it for the bulges, insult it for being too fat, or to achy, or too slow, or too sick. Look disgusted at it when you look in the mirror, and you will have an uncooperative body. Your cells know how you feel about them. They respond to the emotional reactions by changing the chemical and electrical messages that pour through your body. The result is confusion about what to do... fulfill your images of disgust or follow the desires of your heart.

Now, of all the resources you have at hand, this next one may be the most important. That's why I saved it for one of the last parachutes. Grit your teeth and just do it.

1. Stand in front of the mirror, NAKED, and gently stroke your body telling it you appreciate it for the years of service it has given you. (Stick with me, now.) Tell your body that you love it, as it is, NOW.
2. Give your body unconditional love and acceptance, just as you would like for yourself from others. In the light of that love, your body will feel nurtured, accepted and will be eager to cooperate with you.
3. Your body has less than optimal health now because you have fought it and failed to nurture it with kindness and appreciation. Now you are going to take this outcast back into your life with gratitude and love. Stroke every part of your body and give it the loving attention it has gone without for so long.

Cooperation is gained through love, not disgust. You'll be amazed how this attitude-change will make life so much more enjoyable. Every morning when you are getting dressed, take the time to love your body, AS IT IS, NOW, letting it know you are doing your best to treat it right in the best way you know how, from now on.

BELIEFS AND SELF-TALK

PARACHUTE #17

Releasing limited beliefs.
Discovering the creator within.
Owning your Self.

Our unconscious mind holds all of our beliefs, even though most of them are hidden from our conscious mind, buried in layers of experience and forgotten, ever-changing memories. Some of the most powerful beliefs that are controlling our life experience, right now, were placed into the vault of our unconscious mind by parents, siblings, relatives, teachers, and religious leaders when we were too young to analyze them. Up to the age of seven or eight, we simply accepted those words, comments, and teachings as gospel truth because our brain was still incapable of discernment.

Today, we wonder why we sometimes feel stuck, desiring our lives to be different, yet seemingly unable to achieve our dreams.

SOME EARLY MESSAGES CONTROLLING OUR LIVES

- ✓ "Be careful."
- ✓ "Don't take risks."
- ✓ "You're not lovable."
- ✓ "You're not smart, or pretty, or outgoing enough."
- ✓ "You have to prove your manhood."
- ✓ "It has to be perfect."
- ✓ "God is watching you."
- ✓ "You should take care of everyone."
- ✓ "There's not enough to go around."
- ✓ "You should put others before yourself."
- ✓ "You're selfish."
- ✓ "You're no good."
- ✓ "You're always late."
- ✓ "You'll never be good enough to ...."

SOME MORE EARLY MESSAGES CONTROLLING OUR LIVES

- ✓ "You can't afford it."
- ✓ "You're a sinner."
- ✓ "You're a wimp."
- ✓ "It's too much for you."
- ✓ "Life is tough."
- ✓ "You'll never amount to anything."
- ✓ "Boys should be strong and never show emotions."
- ✓ "Girls need daddy to take care of them."
- ✓ "You gotta work hard for everything."
- ✓ "Nothing comes easy."
- ✓ "Money is everything."
- ✓ "Money corrupts."
- ✓ "Always be nice."
- ✓ "Don't talk back."
- ✓ "The end is worth the means, no matter what."

ADD YOUR OWN

_____
_____
_____
_____
_____
_____
_____
_____
_____
_____
_____
_____
_____
_____
_____

The point is, these statements that were placed into our unconscious minds were just statements. They were coming from the minds of others and they didn't really have anything to do with us. In other words, …

They are not and never were true.

Whenever you find yourself thinking negative and "I can't" thoughts, immediately stop and ask yourself if they are really true for you. Where did that thought come from? Do you WANT to believe it? If you don't want to believe it, then don't.

CHANGE THE BELIEFS THAT NO LONGER SERVE YOUR BEST INTERESTS.

Beliefs are not set in stone except if you believe they are, and that's only a belief, as well. Our present and our future are created by what we believe. How do you see yourself in the future? If you see and imagine yourself with poor health and problems in life, you will find that to be exactly what you will experience. *You are always right.*

If you see and FEEL yourself as well, whole, experiencing goodness and happiness in your life, you will experience that because *you are always right.*

We are what we believe. We create what we are thinking about and expecting in our life. If you don't like what is occurring in your life, check out what you are saying to yourself. "I feel so bad." "I'm afraid it won't work out." "There isn't enough time." "Something might go wrong." And the big one, "I'm too old."

No, no, no. Don't go there anymore. We kill ourselves with our don'ts and doubts. Our biggest trap is fear. Fear begets exactly what we fear. Belief gets us what we believe.

CHOOSE TO BE HEALTHY, HAPPY AND WHOLE
THEN LIVE YOUR LIFE AS IF THAT WERE TRUE FOR YOU RIGHT NOW.

Regardless of your life circumstances at this moment, know that they are a product of your past thinking. From this moment forward, decide what your future will be. Choose the best.

To assist you with creating your desired future I recommend the books and tapes by Dr. Wayne Dyer. *Excuses Begone!* and *Wishes Fulfilled.* Read or listen to the tapes/DVDs over and over. They can change your life and they will, if you let them.

BELIEFS I AM CHOOSING NOW TO CREATE THE FUTURE I DESIRE

"I am visualizing and feeling these beliefs to be true for me right now."

A PERSONAL MESSAGE

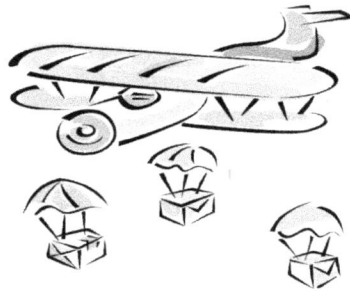

"I wish you success because you were created to have optimal health and you are capable of achieving much more than you are aware of. I wish for you, profound peace of mind and happiness in life. I send you my love, understanding and sincere caring. I share your tears of joy as you release all that is holding you back and you discover the real you, body, mind and spirit, inside. You have all the inner resources you need to create your dreams and make them come true. Determine to have optimal health, use your resources, believe in yourself, and you will achieve it." Dr. Suka

"If you have the faith of a grain of mustard seed,
nothing shall be impossible for you."
Matthew 17:20

LET YOUR SPIRIT SOAR

APPENDIX

APPENDIX A

VIOLENCE AND MENTAL ILLNESS –
WHO'S AT FAULT?

We acknowledge there are several explanations for the increase in national violence including violence on TV, breakup of families, absence of a good education, and growing poverty. Guns, however, are not responsible for violence any more than cars are responsible for drunk drivers. It's the shooter we need to look at. Significantly, there is one explanation that the media and others are not addressing.

LEGAL DRUG PUSHING

An increase in medicating the mind with psychotic drugs has provoked a crisis in mental health with appalling consequence: mass killings by our youth.[1]

Between 2004-2011 there were almost thirteen thousand reports to the FDA's Med Watch system of psychiatric drugs causing violent side effects, suggesting that the side effects from these drugs are nine or ten times higher than admitted in official data.

In an analysis of mass shootings during the past fifteen years, *every shooter had been taking or withdrawing from a psychiatric drug*. In these thirty-one school shootings or school-related acts of violence, one hundred sixty-two were wounded and seventy-two were killed.[2]

Peter Breggin, MD, psychiatrist, notes that, "One of the things in the past that we've known about depression is that it very, very rarely leads to violence. It's only been since the advent of these new SSRI drugs that we've had murderers, even mass murders, taking these antidepressant drugs." According to Breggin, "psychiatric drugs can cause or worsen violence" in those who take them and cites a 2010 study of reports to the FDA on drug-induced violence which has demonstrated that antidepressants have resulted in an 840% increase in the rate of violence among those taking the drugs.[3]

The answer is to "say no" to these dangerous drugs. Having read this book, you already know there are safe and effective alternatives that address the underlying cause of depression and mental disorders. Inform, inform, inform everyone who will listen. Say "goodbye" to physicians who refuse to budge from pharmaceutical pep talks.

STANDARD AMERICAN DIET (SAD) = MENTAL ILLNESS AND VIOLENCE

Above all, the most influential factor in the course of increasing violence has been changes in the American food system and loss of nutrients for children and growing teens.[4] Listed here are a few examples of nutritional deficiencies or excesses and related associations.

- ✓ Low Vitamin B1 (thiamine) = irritability, sensitive to criticism, aggression
- ✓ Low Vitamin B3 (niacin) = anxiety, hyperactivity, hallucinations, schizophrenic symptoms
- ✓ Low Vitamin B6 (pyridoxine) = irrational anger, psychiatric disorders leading to violence, hallucinations
- ✓ Low Vitamin B5 (pantothenic acid) = hypoglycemia induced aggression, suicide
- ✓ Low Vitamin C = leads to increased copper
- ✓ Excess Copper = extreme fear, paranoia, hallucinations, schizophrenia, bipolar disorder, violence in children and youth
- ✓ Low Magnesium = aggression, schizophrenia
- ✓ Low zinc = hypoglycemia induced suicide, angry, aggressive, hostile behaviors, violence
- ✓ Low DHA (a fatty acid) = violence
- ✓ Food sensitivities = psychotic, schizophrenic symptoms
- ✓ Aspartame & MSG = paranoia, behavioral disorder, schizophrenia (As of this writing the dairy industry is petitioning the FDA to approve aspartame in milk)
- ✓ Over 4000 chemicals are classified as food additives.
- ✓ Food coloring includes lead.
- ✓ Red candies contain aluminum.
- ✓ Diets high in sugar and refined carbohydrates account for most of antisocial behavior, agitation, depression, anger, anxiety, panic attacks and violent behavior.
- ✓ Homicidal offenders have lower cholesterol levels than other criminals.
- ✓ Studies show an association between low cholesterol and deaths due to accidents and violence.
- ✓ Violent suicide attempts are related to lower cholesterol levels than cholesterol levels of non-violent suicides.
- ✓ Soda is linked to violence which increases as levels of soda increase.
- ✓ Coffee includes 300 other chemicals.
- ✓ Caffeine at high doses triggers mania or psychosis.
- ✓ Average baby on a soy-based formula = equates to 5 birth control pills a day containing estrogen and progesterone hormones
- ✓ Soy infant formula creates zinc imbalance = aggression, violent behavior in later years.
- ✓ Soy is washed in aluminum tanks & absorbs aluminum.
- ✓ School lunch programs use 30% soy to meet protein standards = antisocial behavior
- ✓ Prison food includes 40% soy = antisocial behavior
- ✓ Sugar consumption in 1800 = less than 10 pounds. Sugar consumption now = 150 lbs year
- ✓ Hypoglycemia (low blood sugar) = 30-70% psychiatric patients
- ✓ Children fed high amounts of apple juice are at risk for failure to thrive.

VACCINATIONS AND BRAIN INFLAMMATION

Few European countries have mandatory vaccination programs. American children, following the CDC vaccination schedule, receive over thirty-five shots before grade school including twelve shots in the first six months of life. Six of these vaccines contain formaldehyde, five contain a mercury-derivative preservative banned by the FDA in over-the-counter drugs, and another five vaccines contain aluminum leading to developmental disabilities, violent behavior, permanent brain damage and more.

ENVIRONMENTAL TOXINS

1. Blood samples from newborns show exposure to over 287 toxins, including mercury, fire retardants, pesticides and Teflon – exposure that occurs even before they are born. Of these, 180 cause cancer in humans or animals, 208 cause birth defects or abnormal development in animal tests, and 217 are toxic to the brain and nervous system.
2. Heavy metal exposure compromises normal brain development and neurotransmitter function leading to long-term deficits in learning and social behavior.
3. Studies show that hyperactive children and criminal offenders have significantly elevated levels of lead, manganese, or cadmium compared to controls.
4. High blood levels of lead at age seven predict juvenile delinquency and adult crime. Lead is associated with aggressive behavior, crime, juvenile delinquency and behavioral problems.
5. Silicofluorides in the water supply are associated with higher rates of learning disabilities, ADHD, violent crime and criminals using cocaine at the time of arrest. These fluorides increase the amount of lead in the water.
6. Manganese toxicity has a known association with impulsive and violent behavior. Soy infant formulas have very high levels of manganese

Perhaps lead in the pants of politicians is responsible for their disability to learn. In the end, the consumer calls the shots. Buy right, eat right. Say "no" to mind and mood altering substances. Be heard. It's our right to insist upon what helps and avoid what hurts. Together, we will make a difference.

1. The information in this chapter has be excerpted from an article written by Sylvia Onusic, PhD, CNS, LDN that appeared in the Spring 2013 edition of *Wise Traditions*, a publication of the Weston A. Price Foundation. The journal can be ordered through www.westonaprice.org.
2. The Citizen's Commission on Human Rights International. Another School Shooting, Another Psychiatric Drug? Federal Investigation Long Overdue. July 20, 2012
3. Breggin PR. Psychiatry Has No Answer to Gun Massacres, Progressive Radio Network. December 21, 2012
4. Sylvia Onusic, PhD, CNS, LDN, Spring 2013 edition of *Wise Traditions*, a publication of the Weston A. Price Foundation.

APPENDIX B

RECOVERY RESOURCES

Dr. Suka offers an educational, natural approach to recovery. Clients learn how to determine the underlying cause of their symptoms and how to begin an all natural process of rebalancing their brain chemistry. The goal is for the client to be able to take charge of their healing process free from pharmaceutical medications, as much as possible, and to achieve a healthy, symptom-free recovery.

CONSULTATIONS FOR DEPRESSION AND SYMPTOM RELIEF

Dr. Suka consults with clients beginning with a telephone assessment which includes reviewing laboratory tests, gathering history, and providing written and additional laboratory testing, if needed. Clients are encouraged to work with their healthcare provider to reduce or eliminate medications. An individualized biochemical formula consisting of all natural micronutrients, healthy nutrition, and stress reducing guidelines is developed. Ongoing consultations provide support and adjustments to the protocol, as needed. Dr. Suka's philosophy is to work together with clients, as a team, to create a program they are able to comfortably manage according to their unique lifestyle. To schedule a consultation, go to: www.BrainworksRecovery.com.

DO-IT-YOURSELF ALCOHOL RECOVERY PROGRAM

This program is completely outlined in the book *How to Quit Drinking for Good and Feel Good* by Suka Chapel-Horst, RN, PhD. Motivated, highly functioning individuals can live at home, keep it private, continue normal activities, and recover affordably. Consultations are available as needed. For information go to: www.BrainworksAlcoholRecovery.com.

RESIDENTIAL ALCOHOL TREATMENT & AFTERCARE PROGRAMS

Most of our residential clients have been through other treatment programs, or tried AA, and have relapsed, often several times. They want something different and are highly motivated to do whatever it takes to recover. This program stresses symptom-free recovery versus sobriety. The program uses a biochemical approach combined with other natural modalities. Residents live in the home with Dr. Suka and her husband, David, a recovery coach. For information go to: wwww.AriseAlcoholRecovery.com.

CONCIERGE RESIDENTIAL PROGRAM

Clients decide where they want to do their 30 day residential treatment program. Dr. Suka and David will bring the treatment program to the client at their home or to most any location of the client's choice in the U.S. For information go to: www.AriseAlcoholRecovery.com.

MARIJUANA ADDICTION

Read the book *Cannabinoids – The Hundredth Monkey Cure* by Suka Chapel-Horst, RN, PhD, available on http://www.BrainworksRecovery.com, http://www.Amazon.com, and through national booksellers.

APPENDIX C

RECOMMENDED RESOURCES

LABORATORY TESTING

Direct Health: www.pyroluriatesting.com

A large variety of tests are available from Direct Health including, but not limited to, tests for pyroluria, histamine, copper and zinc. They can be ordered directly by the client, through a healthcare provider or through Dr. Suka. Insurance may cover these tests.

Sanesco Health: www.sanescohealth.com

Sanesco Health offers testing for neurotransmitters and adrenal insufficiency. The tests can be ordered through a healthcare provider or through Dr. Suka. Insurance coverage is available.

Life Extension: www.lef.org

Life Extension offers many tests that are available to the public without a prescription. There is no insurance coverage for these tests.

Vitamin D Council: www.vitamindcouncil.com

Inexpensive and accurate Vitamin D testing. No prescription necessary.

INSURANCE

Be aware that a diagnostic code must be attached to all insurance requests. Some people prefer to pay out-of-pocket in order to avoid having a diagnostic label attached to their medical records, for life.

BIPOLAR DISORDER

<u>True Hope:</u> www.truehope.com

    True Hope offers a natural supplement formula that is well researched and has helped many individuals with this disorder. The book *A Promise of Hope* is available from this web site and I recommend it to anyone wanting help with this disorder. The book can also be ordered from www.BrainworksRecovery.com.

APPENDIX D

ADDITIONAL READING

BASIC READING

Food and Behavior – Barbara Reed Stitt, PhD
This book is a classic. School children, prisoners, and probationers reverse negative and criminal behaviors when their diets change. Many case histories. Provides hope and help.

ALCOHOL ADDICTION

How to Quit Drinking for Good and Feel Good - The NEW Alcoholism Story – Suka Chapel-Horst, RN, PhD. Reward Deficiency Syndrome and a biochemical approach to recovery.

ADD/ADHD

Overload – Attention Deficit Disorder and The Addictive Brain - David Miller & Kenneth Blum, PhD.
The underlying cause and correction for ADD and ADHD symptoms. Dr. Blum discovered the genetic code for the biochemical imbalances he named Reward Deficiency Syndrome.

INTERMEDIATE READING

Natural Highs – Hyla Cass, MD & Patrick Holford.
How to feel good all the time. Easy to read, down-to-earth, how-tos for achieving optimal health. Treats specific health issues. Excellent. Biochemical, nutritional approach.

8 Weeks to Vibrant Health – Hyla Cass, MD and Kathleen Barnes.
Achieve optimal health with this easy to read, complete guide to women's health. Biochemical, nutritional approach.

The Yeast Connection & Women's Health – William G. Crook, MD, Hyla Cass, MD, Elizabeth B. Crook
Understanding and treating Candida.

ADVANCED READING

The Diet Cure – Julia Ross, MA, MFT
Best selling book recently updated. Everything you want to know about maintaining good health. Includes latest amino acid therapies.

Mood Cure – Julia Ross, MA, MFT
Author of *Diet Cure* provides tests and food supplement guide to release depression without medications. Includes amino acid replacement as well as nutritional guidelines for many disorders.

Depression Free Naturally – Joan Mathews Larson, PhD.
Natural resources for health. Indepth explanation of biochemical imbalances. Very complete. Be advised that some of the formulas given are now dated.

BIPOLAR DISORDER

A Promise of Hope – Autumn Stringam
Autumn's personal story of her mother's bipolar disorder and the discovery that she, too, was bipolar. She writes about her recovery with the help of the natural supplement formula her father developed that is helping thousands of individuals. You won't want to put this book down until it's finished.

MEDICINE

The Antidepressant Solution – Joseph Glenmullen, MD
Understand antidepressants and how to safely overcome antidepressant withdrawal and dependence. Includes specific guidelines for tapering off antidepressants, withdrawal symptoms, warnings, dangers, and solutions.

SCIENCE and HEALTH

Anatomy of an Epidemic: Magic Bullets, Psychiatric Drugs, and the Astonishing Rise of Mental Illness in America – Robert Whitaker. The stunning rise of mentally ill Americans due to complicity between doctors and pharmaceutical companies.

Overdosed America The Broken Promise of American Medicine – John Abramson
A tell-all accounting about the pharmaceutical industry's duping and doping of Americans.

Nutrient Power – William J. Walsh, PhD.
How to heal your biochemistry and heal your brain. In-depth science and research behind dysfunctional brain chemistry, mental health disorders and the nutritional approach to recovery.

Nutrition and Physical Degeneration – Weston A. Price, DDS
The original book underlying all nutritional guidelines. It's the bottom line to nutrition and why. Fascinating and powerful reading. Learn from our native and aboriginal peoples.

CD'S

Reward Deficiency Syndrome – The Real Cause of Addictions (36 minutes)
Suka Chapel-Horst, RN, PhD, available at www.BrainworksRecovery.com.

BOOK and DVD POWERPOINT PRESENTATIONS WITH TRANSCRIPTS

by Suka Chapel-Horst, RN, PhD, QMHP available through www.BrainworksRecovery.com

Wellness Simplified – How Food affects Moods, Bodies and Behaviors Book/DVD

Think what you eat doesn't matter? Fast food, junk food, sodas, and pizza are the voices of violence, crime, and suicide, as well as obesity, joint pain, insomnia, anxiety, diabetes, depression, cancer, and *you name it!*

What we eat affects the quality of our lives. Sick and tired of feeling sick and tired? Are children's behaviors getting out of hand? Are school grades going down? It's OK. There's a solution and it's not rocket science.

This little book and DVD can change lives for the better, right now. The solution makes sense and it's doable. Say "goodbye" to moods, sickness, and unwanted behaviors. Say "hello" to good health and happiness.

Say Goodbye to Moods and Depression Book/DVD

The only way to restore optimal health is by deleting poisonous nonfoods and feeding the brain the natural substances from which it is made.

Babies are made from food, not Prozac. After birth, why do we switch from the natural building blocks of life to synthetic pills? We can achieve optimal health when we remove the underlying brain chemical imbalances which lead to the symptoms of moods and depression including insomnia, anxiety, panic reactions, irritability, weight gain, aches and pains, and more.

The good news is that targeted micronutrients and healthy nutrition, along with other holistic methods of healthcare, can reduce or eliminate moods and depression, naturally.

The Real Cause and Solution for Alcohol Addiction, The NEW Alcoholism Story Book/DVD

Alcohol addiction is caused by an inherited and genetically caused imbalance of brain chemistry. It's not caused by a character defect, a moral shortcoming, or by a lack of will power.

Neuroscience and biochemistry have proven, once and for all, that all addictions are biochemically caused. It's time to give up shame, blame, and guilt for a disorder that is biochemically caused.

When dysfunctional brain chemistry is restored to normal, relapse and dry-drunk symptoms are rare. Learn how imbalanced brain chemistry leads to alcoholism and discover the recovery method that has the highest long-term relapse-free recovery rate.

The Gift – A Sound Mind for Life Book/DVD

How to increase mental focus, improve memory, and prevent or delay Alzheimer's. The DVD includes biochemical, nutritional, physical, emotional, and mental resources to minimize and delay the effects of aging. Discover how chronic stress underlies most illness and disease and how to reduce the effects of stress naturally. This is valuable information for any age.

Trick or Treat – What Your Doctor isn't Telling You about Mood Altering Medications Book/DVD

Is your doctor treating you or tricking you? If you are considering taking mood altering medications, are already on them, or want to get off them, you need to know what these medications are really doing to brain chemistry. Be informed in order to make wise decisions. Your emotional and mental life is at stake.

PTSD – Post-Traumatic Stress Disorder, Alternative Resources for Recovery Book/DVD

Addressing biochemical, nutritional, brain wave state, and bioenergy fields is a necessary component to recovery, including the clearing of destructive cellular memories using the latest science of energy psychology.

When counseling and medications have failed to return someone with PTSD to a healthy and happy life, it's time to look at the underlying biochemical cause, including the effects of medications on the brain, and to consider alternative solutions to achieve recovery.

Cannabinoids – The Hundredth Monkey Cure Book/DVD

Cannabinoids have been used to treat ailments for over 5,000 years and could be the most useful remedy ever discovered to treat more than 100 human diseases and conditions. It should be used for preventive healthcare, and as a natural support in our increasingly toxic, carcinogenic environment.

All Book and DVD PowerPoint Presentation are available from
www.BrainworksRecovery.com

APPENDIX E

ABOUT THE AUTHOR

"Dr. Suka" Chapel-Horst, RN, PhD, QMHP, is the founder and director of Brainworks Recovery, an educational training, and consulting practice, Brainworks Alcohol Recovery offering Do-It-Yourself alcohol recovery programs, and *ARISE* Alcohol Recovery, a residential treatment and aftercare program. She is a radio show host, a national speaker, and a consultant for clients, internationally.

Dr. Suka has degrees in Nursing, Business, Human Resources, Ministry, Metaphysics and is an interfaith Ordained Minister. She is also a Master Practitioner of Neuro-Linguistics and an EFT (Emotional Freedom Techniques) Practitioner.

Dr. Suka has been an RN for over 40 years, specializing in the fields of Mental Health, Criminal Justice, Drug Dependency, and Wellness Education in Minnesota, Washington, Colorado and North Carolina.

She was a corporate trainer for 15 years, and President of Personal Growth Foundation, an educational organization that provided training programs to over 80,000 participants nationally.

Dr. Suka created and directed the highly successful *Peers Optimal Health Program* conducted in five centers in Minneapolis and St. Paul, MN. In that program over six hundred participants achieved improved health and weight loss, as well as emotional, mental and spiritual upliftment. Pre-existing medical conditions were decreased or eliminated through a combination of biochemical restoration, energy balancing and psychosocial education.

Dr. Suka has been a ski instructor, a National Ski Patrol First Aid Instructor certified in Mountain and Avalanche Rescue, First Aid Instructor and Disaster Representative for the American Red Cross and Professional Rescue Instructor of Minnesota. She has served as a Victim Advocate for the Boulder, CO Police Department and Chaplain for the Boulder County, CO Sheriff's Department. Dr. Suka was a Hospital Chaplain for Presbyterian Hospital in Denver, CO.

Dr. Suka, her husband David, and their Pomeranian, Peekaboo, travel in their motor home throughout the U.S. giving presentations and workshops.

www.BrainworksRecovery.com
www.AriseAlcoholRecovery.com
www.BrainworksAlcoholRecovery.com